So You Want to Be A Doctor...

So You Want to Be A Doctor...

Stuart C. Zeman, M.D.

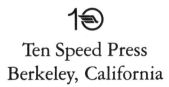

Ten Speed Press
Berkeley, California

🔟

Ten Speed Press
P.O. Box 7123
Berkeley, California 94707

FIRST TEN SPEED PRINTING 1992

Cover design by Fifth Street Design
Author photo by Fisher
Text design by Les Ferriss
Typesetting by Ann Flanagan Typography
Illustrations by Carol Zeman

Library of Congress Cataloging-in-Publication Data

Zeman, Stuart C.
    So you want to be a doctor— / Stuart C. Zeman.
        p.   cm.
    ISBN 0-89815-502-9
    1. Medicine—Vocational guidance.   I. Title.
R690.Z46   1992   92-11876
610.69'52—dc20   CIP

Printed in the United State of America
1   2   3   4   5   —   96   95   94   93   92

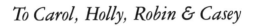

To Carol, Holly, Robin & Casey

Contents

So You Want to Be A Doctor . . .

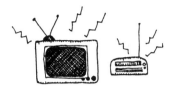

1. Getting Started

THIS IS GREAT. Fourth down and goal and the Packers are going for it. Just hand the ball off to Jimmy Taylor and he'll score. Damn! Another commercial. Oh, well.

"The Niners are driving down the field," blares the radio. If Brodie would just throw simple down-and-out patterns to Parks and Washington, we'd have it made.

Wow! It doesn't get any better than this. One football game on TV and the other on radio. Oh, Christ. He's coming. "Is this how you study, Buck? There is no way in hell you'll get into medical school, or college for that matter, if this is how you study." That was typical of my dad. He hated sports. He never watched sports. He never played sports. He wasn't even coordinated.

I was on the junior high school baseball team for two years. I played second base in the starting lineup, but he never came to a game. All the other parents came. But none of them were doctors.

All of my father's friends seemed weird. Dr. Airhead, the orthopedic surgeon and my father's closest friend, was a real stink bomb. He had the worst B.O.! I never saw the man smile. And he spoke so slowly it was a miracle I didn't fall asleep before he finished talking. At least he was encouraging. "Buck, orthopedics is a fine specialty. You should go into it, especially with your interest in sports."

Dr. Pore was another strange one. He was my dad's dermatology friend. He was five foot one, with Coke-bottle glasses. Every Saturday he rode his expensive French ten-speed bicycle fifteen miles to our house just to make us think he was in good shape. He'd arrive in time for breakfast. Then he'd eat a whole homemade banana cake just because it was free.

"Buck," he'd say, "I remember when I was at Illinois. I studied twenty hours a day. My favorite course was biochemistry. That's why I like dermatology. It deals with cell pathology." I wasn't even sure what that meant. I just knew I didn't want to be like him.

Then there was our neighbor Dr. Jigger, the internist. He had bad breath, but that was because he smoked. I rarely saw the man without a drink in his hand either. He was friendly though. I got the impression from my dad that he wasn't well respected in the community. Probably because he was drunk most of the time.

One day he took me skiing to the Sierras in his silver Ford Mustang. I liked his approach to life. "Why don't you go to medical school where you can ski too?" he asked. Unlike the others, he knew how to have fun and thought it should be part of everyone's life. He wasn't a good skier. Probably because his alcohol level affected his coordination.

He wouldn't just give advice, talk about stuff I didn't understand, or criticize my study habits and my love for sports. He'd ask questions about my intentions in medicine. On the way home, he stopped at his office to get the mail. "Come on in. I'll just be a second," he said. We walked into his suite, and he invited me to sit at his desk while he perused the mail. Then he opened his bottom desk drawer and pulled out a bottle of scotch. "I've had a long day on the slopes, Buck. May as well end it with a little pop," he smiled.

I knew I didn't want to be like these guys, but I always knew I wanted to be a doctor. I grew up knowing I'd be a doctor. There was no question about it. My father was a doctor and his brother was one too.

My dad was intelligent and well educated. He was well respected in the community and got lots of freebies from his patients. "Thanks for making me see again," one of his deli-owning patients said as he gave us another free lunch. My dad was good at fixing eyeballs— ophthalmology, diseases and surgery of the eye.

As the service station owner lubed and oiled my dad's Cadillac for free he said, "My mother lives by herself since you gave her those new glasses. Thanks to you, my wife and I now have a life of our own."

I quickly learned the power of good connections. My older brother was arrested several times when he was a teenager. But my dad knew the judges. Dickie got probation and served no jail time.

Freebies, money, respect, power, independence, and nice cars. Medicine looked like the perfect profession.

The best thing about junior high was Mrs. Robinson, my history teacher. She was a nice piece of work—good-looking, with a terrific pair of legs. Every time she sat down at her desk, she would make sure I was looking at her legs. And I was. She wore dark brown stockings and her legs weren't always held tightly together. When we took tests, she'd stop at my desk and lean over making sure her breasts were touching my shoulder. She had a great body.

Besides history, there was algebra, English, science, and home room. They all seemed worthless to me. "Mental masturbation" was what my dad called it.

I wasn't a part of the "in-crowd" during junior high. I was too busy playing baseball and studying so I could make the grade to get into college. Not just any college either, it had to be the university so it would look good on my record for medical school. It sounded like bull to me but what did I know? I just knew I wanted to be a doctor, so I went along with what my dad told me.

In high school the courses were harder and even more irrelevant than in junior high. German was really a waste. I would memorize phrases for a test and forget them the same day. But I was required to take a foreign language as a prerequisite for entrance into the university.

In chemistry my teacher looked like a flask. His face was pointed. He got his jollies out of pop quizzes. We'd walk into class, put down our books, and as soon as the bell would ring he'd say, "Put everything away, it's time for a quiz." Some asinine way to see if we'd been studying. He was always serious, never cracked a smile. He was dull. I kept saying to myself, is this what I'm in for, just trying to get into medical school? I told myself it was a means to an end. It had to be done.

I was so scared about making the grade to get into the university that I felt guilty about having fun. Most nights the popular people went out on dates and to athletic events. I always felt I should be studying so I could get all A's. Then I could get into medical school and be a doctor. I was repulsed by this recurrent theme in every moment of my life. But I knew what I wanted, so I did what I thought I had to do to get there. My dad led me to believe that I had to study all the time or else I wouldn't get to be a doctor.

I never received positive feedback for my determination. Few people cared that I wanted to be a doctor. My teachers said, "That's admirable, but it's a long haul." Friends said, "Boy, you're really going to make a lot of money." People who knew my parents remarked, "It would be great to follow in your father's footsteps. He worked hard to establish himself and you can carry on the family name."

To make the grade in high school, I had to set aside my athletic desires. My father would not allow me to go out for football because it took too much time away from studying. Even if I could have afforded the time, I would have been too tired to study when I got home at night. And, of course, the statistics. They showed that eighty percent of people who played tackle football suffered some permanent disability. "Look here, it's in this medical journal," my dad said. "Read it for yourself. You can read, can't you? If you can't, you'll never get into medical school," he said time and again.

Well, how about the golf team? It was not strenuous. I wouldn't be tired when I got home, and I would only play a couple of months out of the year. What a compromise. But golf wasn't enough exercise for me. Finally, my dad agreed to let me continue playing baseball. I was relieved by this decision since most of my friends were athletes and I couldn't relate to bookworms.

"Son, why don't you get a summer job at the hospital? You could be an orderly in the emergency room," my dad suggested. What a dumb idea. I worked my ass off all year long in the classroom and I didn't want to work in a hospital being pushed around by a bunch of stiff nurses telling me to empty bedpans. Would that be good experience? Did it pay worth a damn? No. I didn't need to be in a hospital. I knew what a hospital smelled like—an alcohol swab.

My idea of a summer job was to air out my brain, use it as little as possible, and make a lot of money. I found the perfect job working for a neighbor who managed a local can company. He was a big boozer, but he liked kids. He gave several of us jobs. In the one-hundred-degree heat, we repaired bins for shipping tomatoes from the field to the cannery. These bins were usually damaged by some hung-over forklift driver who had loaded them improperly. The good thing about the job was that it forced me to be in great shape and the pay was fantastic. I earned at least three times what my friends were earning.

After I repaired bins for about six weeks, I was moved to the weighmaster position. This job was the best of all. I sat at the weigh station for twelve to fourteen hours a day watching T.V., waiting for trucks to drive across the scale so I could weigh them. That took about five minutes. From there they went through inspection and off to the cannery. I had my own phone so I could talk to my friends whenever I wanted.

Normally, after three days I had accumulated over forty hours and everything after that was paid at time and a half. As incredible as it sounds, I earned union wages without having to join the union, because it was just a summer job. My paychecks were so big that within two summers I had earned enough to pay for the majority of my college and medical education.

Paying for my education was important to me. I didn't want to be beholden to anybody in case things didn't work out or I didn't make the grade. But if I did, I wanted to be able to say that I had done it myself and I owed no one. I knew it would bug me if my father said, "Yes, we put Buck through school so he would have time to study, and he wouldn't have to worry about working part-time to pay for his books."

One summer I stayed with my uncle from Illinois. He was not like the other doctors. He worked hard but he played hard too. He usually did three to four surgeries in a morning and then, in the afternoon, he drove his fancy Buick to the country club and played golf. I really liked the fact that he wasn't afraid to spend money and enjoy himself.

My uncle was a great guy, but the work he did was sure nauseating. In the early years of cancer surgery, he was one of the foremost authorities on tumors of the jaw and face. He would remove one side of a face and turn up a large flap of skin from the shoulder to cover the area eaten by the tumor. No matter if one side of the face was hairless and the other your armpit. It was necessary. Aren't doctors suppose to save lives, prolong health, and stamp out disease?

He always liked me because I wanted to go to medical school. Frequently he would invite me to his meetings. These guys weren't stupid either. They would go to nice spots, like Pebble Beach or Palm Springs, where they could lecture in the morning and play golf in the afternoon.

The bad part was that I had to listen to the exact same lectures every time I went. After two or three of these, I could have given them myself. "Here is a seventy-five-year-old female with a malignant osteosarcoma of the jaw. She is five years postoperative and is feeling great. Repeat tests show that there is no recurrence of the tumor." True, but at Halloween she needs no costume.

He often told me, "If you don't get into medical school in California, I can easily get you into a school here, since I carry a lot of clout in Illinois." He was a full professor of otorhinolaryngology (ear, nose, and throat—ENT) at two Illinois universities. He also claimed to have friends at another Chicago medical school and almost anyone could buy their way into that institution. I could have my choice. Pick the one most suited to my study habits and all of them would prepare me nicely to go into otorhinolaryngology.

Ah, but wait a minute. Who said I wanted to go into ENT? Did I want to look up noses every day? Did I want to slide my way past mounds of ear wax to look at some screaming child's eardrum? Did I want to peer down some phlegm-filled throat to see if I could snare a chicken bone that had been inadvertently swallowed?

I didn't want to disappoint him and I didn't want to lose my Illinois connection, so I kept my mouth shut. As it turned out, I was inept at using the light mirror to peer down the throats of patients, so I could never have made it in ENT. I was always trying to adjust my neck rather than the mirror. Finally, once I got the mirror adjusted, the patient would cough in my face and fog the mirror.

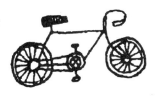

2. College

I FINALLY got into college, despite my father's comments about my poor study habits. And not just any college, I made it into the university. My dad said I was among the elite, one of the few students who had made the grade, the best of the best. I didn't have good grades by premedical standards but I squeaked by, my way. I chose Aggie University, only a fifteen-mile drive each weekend from a home-cooked meal and the washing machine. My mother found the new white sheets repulsively discolored when I brought them home every three months. But she never criticized me. She constantly reassured me I would succeed. She was terrific.

College began with a week-long orientation. I familiarized myself with the large lecture halls, the stuffy science laboratories, and the sterile dormitory where I would be living. Basically I went to get acquainted with my prison cell for the next four years.

In the dorms, in the bookstore, everywhere I went, it seemed like everyone was pre-med. "Hi, I'm Jack. I'm from Monterey. I'm pre-med." "Hello, I'm Jennifer. I'm from L.A. and couldn't decide on a major, so I'm pre-med."

Nine out of ten students I met were pre-med. These weren't to be my friends. They just represented pressure and competition. I hated them. I went into the men's room and saw that someone had written, "Hi, I'm Mike, what's your major?" I wrote, "I'm Ding-Dong and I'm pre-med."

The majors you could select to be pre-med were very flexible. You could choose zoology, biology, chemistry, calculus, or botany. Or would you liked to be hanged by the neck until dead?

The first year of college was as much fun as sitting in an electric chair. Lectures were filled with about 250 pimple-faced students with four pencils in their breast pockets and large erasers and thick pads of yellow paper on their desks. Everyone wore glasses and reminded me of Dr. Pore, my father's friend who told me he had studied twenty hours a day to get into medical school. These bookworms were my competition. I was screwed. Not many of us sat in the back where we could sleep unnoticed. We all knew if we got a bad grade, we'd have trouble getting into medical school. There were a limited number of medical school slots and too many pre-med students.

As a science major, sixteen units allowed me the privilege of taking twenty-five hours of classes each week. In contrast, my friend, an economics major with sixteen units, had only sixteen hours of class. He took such biggies as economics, philosophy, and logic. Sounds tough, I know. But that was fair because he would not be able to be called Doctor someday. Instead he would just have to settle for Chief Financial Officer or Chairman of the Board.

I had hoped that living in the dorms would be a socially rewarding experience. Not for me. I didn't have time. I had two goals, to earn good grades and to make the university baseball team.

I went to college six weeks early to begin baseball tryouts. Some days we would practice twice a day just to get in shape. One hundred fifty guys went out for the team. Only thirty of us made it.

Once school began, we practiced each day for three hours, usually between 3:00 and 6:00 p.m. As a pre-med student, I had chemistry labs that went from 1:00 to 4:00 p.m., but my instructors allowed me to leave early on the condition that I return by 7:00 to finish the experiment. But wait. When did I eat dinner? I ate a big breakfast and lunch. Dinner consisted of sunflower seeds on the baseball diamond.

I wanted to do what the rest of my friends were doing, like "party." But I didn't have time.

I was athletic and rowdy. My roommate was plump and religious. I taught him some choice words and he taught me some choice prayers. He left every weekend for religious retreats while I headed home with my duffel bag. The dorms were too noisy to study there on weekends. So much for the college experience outside the classroom.

Though the dorms resembled the nearby state penitentiary, they were close to campus and I didn't have to cook. In the dining hall we would talk about the day's lectures and those tenured professors who could lecture for sixty minutes straight without ever looking up at the class.

The university was big on the tenure system, rewarding all the academic freeloaders with a signed contract for life. What did they do? They taught one class a quarter. The teaching assistants graded all the papers and did the research. It was important for these parasites to have free time so they could leave their offices by 10:30 a.m. and head out to the Aggie Airport. Many of them had their pilot's licenses and belonged to the Flying Aggies Club, which rented them a plane for luncheon trips to the Almond Patch Restaurant and Airport.

They did this with such regularity that no flight plan was necessary. After a brief inspection of the plane, they took off for the fifteen-minute flight to the Almond Patch. After touchdown around 11:30, allowing for abnormal wind conditions (like their lectures), they took a small choo-choo train from the airport to the restaurant for cocktails followed by lunch. Cocktails? Wasn't that against federal regulations, to drink within eight hours of flying? Who did they think they were, commercial airline pilots?

Later, as a medical student, I was taken on this trip. I was even allowed to pay for the meal, since it was in vogue to take your professor to lunch. Especially if you wanted to be damn sure to pass your tests.

When the professors finished lunch, around 1:30 or 2:00 p.m., they would fly back to make sure they were in their offices no later than 3:00. Do the taxpayers feel nauseated yet?

The large classrooms all emptied out for lunch at the same time. At least one thousand students mounted their bicycles. (It was still too early in the year to be mounting each other.) This was an orthopedic surgeon's delight. People would crash into each other and get hurt. Even if a co-ed just skinned her knee, there were eight guys shouting, "Don't worry, I'm pre-med!"

Sometimes I couldn't find my bicycle, something every student had for transportation on this large, level campus. I thought the famous Aggie Honor System had failed. It was not unusual to see a bike chained to a tree with links bigger than anchors. But I eventually found mine among the others. I used the principle that if you rode a clunker, a bike that looked and sounded like a complete wreck, no one would steal it. This worked for the entire six years I spent at Aggie University.

I always looked forward to lunch. This was my time to relax. I could go to the quad, sit on the grass, and listen to the protesters scream over the public address system about Vietnam. Many were non-students who smoked pot and danced to the band that sometimes played. Here I was, trying to read biochemistry, and the music was so loud that the ice was rattling in my Coke.

I would have gone to the dorm for lunch, but I didn't like eating with my roommate. He always sat across from me and chewed with his mouth open. It was like peering into a cement mixer.

The dorm food was a daily adventure. Swiss steak tasted like cat food. Eggs were like bubble gum, gravy like sulfuric acid. The only good thing was that dorm residents worked part-time checking people in at the door. Most of them were our friends and didn't care who we brought with us. We'd take our buddies from off-campus housing to eat at our Cafe Dormitoree. The price was right. As my mom said, "Such a deal."

My grades were okay the first year. I didn't get all A's, but I only got one C. Of course my dad said those grades would not be good enough to get me into the medical school of my choice, but hopefully I could get in somewhere—like Guadalajara.

I was in constant motion my freshman year, but I had a good time. I especially enjoyed getting out of chemistry lab at 5:30 p.m., just in time to see my economics and philosophy major friends playing intramural sports or lying out by the pool as I was returning to my room to study. But that was okay, I was going to be a doctor. And once I got into medical school, took an internship, completed a five-year residency, and took the Boards, it would be worth it. Horse manure.

By my second year I quit the baseball team. I needed more time to study. Besides, going to parties and dating were looking better than baseball.

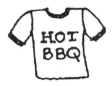

3. Applying to Medical School

DURING my third year of college, I began the lengthy process of applying to medical schools. Did this mean I was starting to see the light at the end of the tunnel? Well, not really. But it made me feel like I was making progress. Maybe I'd be able to wear a white coat soon and feel like a real doctor. When medical students go to class, they get to wear white coats, don't they? Maybe not.

Where do I apply? The advice from my father was, "Apply to as many schools as possible. Hopefully you'll have a few choices. Preferably apply to those in California so you won't be charged out-of-state tuition." My uncle in Chicago told me to apply to schools in Illinois because I would be a shoo-in with his connections. He said, "I might have to make a few phone calls, but it would be no problem. Count on it."

My college advisor said, "Apply to the schools where you want to live." I thought he was the most naive. The medical school underground, among the pre-med students, knew which schools were supposedly the easiest to get into. Everyone agreed that the more schools applied to, the better your chances.

My thoughts were to apply to the least expensive schools. I wanted to be able to say I put myself through medical school. Sounds macho, I know.

So I sent for all the applications. It only cost a stamp and I wrote a form letter to each school saying I wanted to apply to their most prestigious institution. In a few weeks, I received a bunch of thick envelopes and began the tedious process of filling in the endless amount of information.

I got tired of the same questions over and over and wanted to have some fun. One school back East required a $200 application fee. That was too expensive, so I decided not to send the money, but to answer the questions in ways I really wanted. On the question about my parents' occupations, I wrote that my father was a drug dealer and my mother a prostitute. "But don't worry," I wrote, "I turned out okay."

The application asked if I saw any relationship between running a student body campaign and setting up a medical office. I explained that they were similar because in both you made promises that you knew you couldn't keep. You used as many favors as possible, and when in office, you forgot all of your promises and started stepping on people to climb to the top. And you always smiled. You couldn't be successful in politics or in medicine unless you acquired one of those insincere grins that said, I'm delighted to meet you and how can I use you? I changed my name and mailed the application. Such fun. And all for just a stamp.

Another favorite question was, "Have you ever applied to medical school before?" I always wanted to write that this was my eighth year of applying to your beloved school, but each time I came for an interview, the zits on my face were draining so excessively the interviewer was offended.

I also liked it when they asked me to list all of my extracurricular activities. I was never in any of those clicky clubs but listed them just for fun because I knew the schools never checked. I boasted I had been president of the school glee club, student body treasurer, a local representative to the National 4-H Club, team captain of the varsity basketball team, editor of the school newspaper, and student body advisor to the principal. Before each interview, I had to review my application so I could comment on these worthwhile activities and how they would help contribute to my future as a physician.

Probably the best joke of the entire medical school application process was the question, "Why do you want to become a doctor?" All of the standard reasons were a big bore and didn't even sound good in interviews. For example, I want to help people, I like solving people problems, and I'm good in science. Or my father is a doctor and I want to follow in his footsteps and take over his practice. All of these reasons were wonderful, but had been seen on millions of applications. Committee members longed for something different.

I wrote that I wanted to go into orthopedic surgery because I had always liked carpentry. I got excited at the thought of an athlete blowing out the ligaments in his knee so I could put them back together. Orthopedics is bones, screws, and hammers. The ligaments shatter, needing to be rebuilt and reassembled.

I explained that I had considered becoming a sculptor and Dr. Airhead had told me that a good cast should look like a sculpture. In orthopedic surgery I could mold a plaster of paris cast in the shape of a thigh bone or carve the most beautiful definition out of a short leg cast. Granted, the people reading this thought I was full of shit, but it separated me from the rest of the bookworms.

Letters of recommendation were key. You generally needed two from professors and two from family and friends who could speak to your moral and ethical character. I strived to find professors who would write something out of the ordinary.

I got my zoology professor to write a letter about the human anatomical specimens I had prepared. He bragged how he had never seen a student spend so much time into the wee hours of the morning playing with the little muscles and fingers until they seemed to dance to my voice. These specimens, which I chemically dried, cured, and painted, were part of the donated body program, which allowed me to do the project. The specimens are still used at the medical school for teaching purposes.

During my residency I used one of the specimens while testifying in a superior court case. When the defense attorney asked if I could demonstrate to the jury exactly how an ankle was injured by a revolving door, I whipped out one of my specially prepared legs from a grocery bag. The appalled judge nearly climbed under the bench.

Another letter I cherished was from my chemistry professor, who bragged, "Buck was one of my better chemistry students. He always had a flare for excitement in the laboratory." He never figured out how I dumped a potent solution on the workbench, dissolving all of my lab papers and part of my bench, and still came up with the exact answer on the experiment.

Then there was the time I ignited three test tubes, which started a major fire in the lab. I quickly regained my composure, extinguished the fire, and finished my experiment. The professor amusingly recalled that the graduate student who was our lab instructor was last seen bolting out the door. He never returned to teaching.

Once you mailed all the applications and begged those providing personal references to send in the letters on time, you sat back in anticipation. There were several potential letters you could receive. The school could send a form letter saying your application was being processed and as soon as the appropriate reviews were made, they would be in touch. Another letter could say your application was complete and, pending a review of all applications (so they could see how many were better than yours), they would contact you. Still another letter stated that they would like to arrange for an interview and gave you the choice of one date. No one was ever accepted without an interview.

Finally, my favorite form letter was this:

Dear Mr. Mays:

Thank you so much for your interest in the Knife Happy School of Medicine. As you know, we receive thousands of applications for just a few openings at our famous medical institution. Each year we have the impossible task of choosing the best candidates.

Unfortunately, this year we had an excessive number of qualified students and we are afraid we cannot offer you a position in next year's class. However, we very much appreciate your special interest in the Knife Happy School of Medicine and we sincerely hope that this rejection will in no way discourage your medical endeavors. Thank you very much for your interest.

Sincerely,

Dr. I. Skruyu
Dean of Admissions

Can you imagine how I felt after getting a few of these gems? Granted, many of my attempts were shots in the dark, but how could schools write simple letters like that after I had spent many hours filling out all that crap? Oh well, it was their loss. How were they to know at that stage of my development that I would eventually wear a championship football ring and be considered one of the best technicians in my field?

Luckily, I was invited on several interviews. They presented several problems, especially the ones out of state. First, I missed several days of classes. Occasionally I tried to combine several interviews on what I called a "tour of schools." Second, it was expensive to fly across country, stay overnight, and get meals and ground transportation. Multiply this several times and I had blown a considerable wad.

I could have asked my parents to help, but then I would have had to justify why I was traveling to Boston when there were numerous medical schools within one hundred miles in California. They didn't understand that the classes in Boston were larger or that the average grade point of last year's California class was 3.9. It was easier to go into debt, and this expense would turn out to be virtually nothing when I started to accumulate "real" debt from medical school.

When it was time for my interview, there were a few obvious things to remember. I looked my best. If someone interviewed me who was hung up on being well dressed, I didn't want to disappoint him after I had traveled three thousand miles.

I made sure I was prompt. Even if I had to arrive a half day early. I knew to allow for plane cancellations and other screw-ups by the transportation geniuses of the world. Remember at all times: the airlines don't care about you. They cancel flights on a whim.

If I missed the interview, I might never get another one, or if I did, it could be several weeks or even months later. By then, many of the openings would have been filled, which would lessen my chance for admission.

I always reviewed a copy of my application to be familiar with the lies I had written. Finally, during the interview, I was polite and humble. This nonsense that I knew I was one of the best students to apply to the school, or that several schools had already accepted me, never cut it.

I found it helpful to familiarize myself with the area where I was headed. It seemed inevitable that the interviewer would ask, "Why do you want to come to Chicago?" I was ready. I said, "Since I was born in Chicago, I have always been a Cubs fan. I lived and breathed Ernie Banks and Billy Williams as a kid. I admired the Wrigley family for standing up to political pressure about the lights on the baseball field."

When I went to Washington, D.C., I said to the professor, "I could spend hours at the Smithsonian Institute just learning about American history. Chills went down my spine when I stood in front of the Lincoln Memorial." Incidentally, I didn't get into either of these schools.

Some of the other questions I was asked really surprised me and that was not easy to do. One professor asked, "What do you think about admitting minorities who might not be academically qualified into this medical school?" I responded, "Every person in the country deserves medical care. Since the distribution of physicians across this great land of ours is inadequate in deprived areas, maybe minorities would be more sensitive about returning to their birthplaces to help the needy."

I was very impressed with my answer on the spur of the moment. It was really a shame I couldn't be more honest, especially when I knew that some qualified student was going to take the shaft by a minority being admitted in his place. Statistics clearly documented that, upon graduation, minorities were no more likely to return to deprived areas than the rest of us. They all headed for the same metropolitan and affluent areas that were nice places to live. But remember, say what they want to hear, not what you feel. Incidentally, I got into that school. Not as a minority, smart ass!

It never hurt to get to the interview early to have a chat with the interviewer's secretary. It's the old adage: "Get to the secretary and you get to the boss." One of the schools I applied to in the South was such a case. I arrived at my interview about ninety minutes early and the shapely secretary asked me if I would like a cup of coffee or if I wanted to walk around the campus. She was too nice. Normally secretaries were tired of applicants and they treated us like we had the plague. Or they would just say, "Wait outside until we call you."

But this lady had the sweetest Southern accent and was very friendly. She wanted to know about my trip. When she heard I was from California, she mentioned her brother, who turned out to live only thirty minutes from me. It was suggested that I might want to go out and get some lunch, as the interviewer would be an hour late.

I told her I longed for some hot Southern barbeque because I couldn't get the "good stuff" back in California. I asked for directions to such a restaurant. She mentioned a great place, but the directions were quite complicated. Laughingly, she told me I probably wouldn't find it. I told her I felt a little funny asking, but I would be honored if she would join me since it was the lunch hour and I was buying. She looked around the office to see if anyone was listening. When she accepted my offer, I knew I was in. I could see my acceptance letter.

At lunch we talked about the silly admissions process. I felt great when she talked about all the stuffy applicants that had been interviewed in the past two weeks. She laughed when I spilled the barbeque sauce on my tie.

We returned and her boss showed up even later than expected. At this point I didn't care. I felt good about the situation and good about the school. The interview went well even though the chairman reiterated how famous the school was and how difficult it was to get in. He said my chances were slim since I was from out of state. I sensed he liked me, but I think it was mainly because we talked about golf for most of the interview and he discovered I was a good "stick." When he mentioned his handicap, I said it sounded like he was an excellent golfer and that he belonged to what I had heard was a very prominent country club.

As I left, the secretary gave me a great smile and said, "See you next year." After I left I had the cab driver stop at the barbeque place where we had had lunch. I picked up one of the large red T-shirts displaying the name of the restaurant on the front. When I returned home, I sent the T-shirt to the secretary by Federal Express. I was accepted two weeks later. This, my friends, is how the world goes around.

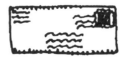

4. Acceptance to Medical School

I REMEMBER when I received my first acceptance letter to medical school. I was at my parents' house because my dirty laundry had built up to alarming proportions. The white sheets had once again turned pale brown. All of my medical school correspondence was sent to my folks' house because mail sent to the dormitory had a way of getting lost. And these medical school applications were my whole life. Or so I thought at the time.

I was chatting with our neighbor while waiting for the mailman to arrive. The mailman was friendly, but the poor guy was tired of my constantly hounding him about possible letters from medical schools. He felt threatened when he showed up without something for me. He had learned that a small envelope probably indicated a rejection and a larger one meant something good, like an acceptance or perhaps more forms to be completed.

On this day he seemed to be in a particular hurry. I had never seen a mail truck burn rubber before. He nearly sideswiped a pickup truck as he left one house and headed toward ours. As he approached, he had a big grin on his face and said, "Big envelope, Doctor." He nervously waited. My heart began to pound. Our neighbor cringed. I had the whole damn block so shook up over this, it was pitiful.

I ripped open the large manila envelope and removed a packet of papers. The cover letter was not a form letter. This, in itself, was a good sign. I read aloud, "It is with great pleasure that I inform you of your acceptance to the Aggie University School of Medicine." My entire body went into spasm. I had done the impossible. The marginal student, who could not concentrate and who had the worst possible study habits, had been accepted into medical school. The dingbat, who watched one game on television while listening to another on radio, had broken into the academic elite.

I hugged the mailman and in the process nearly turned over his little truck. My neighbor picked up a handful of freshly cut grass out of the street pile and threw it high into the air. The postman honked his less than impressive horn. Hearing all the fuss, my father walked out of the garage. As he studied the letter, a tear dropped from his eye. We had done it.

During the next hour, the entire block realized it was safe to come out. There was, in fact, no homicide in the area. We popped a bottle of champagne as everyone, including the mailman, began to call me my lifelong dream, "Doctor."

I spent the day on "Cloud Nine." Even if no other schools accepted me, I had gotten into one and that was all it took. I wanted to tell the world. I quickly canceled all plans to study and embarked on numerous routes to inform my friends. I rushed to the local ice cream store where I had spent many hours over a milk shake wondering if this day would ever come. I wanted to buy ice cream for all the customers, but the owner was so happy, and probably in such disbelief, he bought cones for everyone.

God, was this wonderful! It had finally paid off—all of the bad grades that had threatened my self-esteem, and missing out on all of the fun things the other kids got to do. Maybe I still had a long way to go and maybe my studying was only beginning. But in a sense it was over. I had won. I felt as if I had just hit a home run in the bottom of the ninth with two outs and the bases loaded.

As it turned out, over the next two months I received two more acceptances. Of course they were not nearly as climactic. But it still felt good because now I had a choice. The schools were clearly different. I had been accepted to a state school, close to home and friends, with low tuition. Another was a Chicago school with high tuition, weather cold enough to freeze your nards, and close only to a few relatives. And then there was the academically oriented Southern school, far from home, with cold weather and high tuition. But with a great secretary. Obviously, number one should and did win.

For once in my life, school became fun. Oh sure, I still had to study and make decent grades, but unless I totally decompensated, I was in. I no longer had to look at the pre-med students in my class wishing they would drop dead so I could get a place in medical school. I no longer had to avoid talking to people in case they had been accepted and I hadn't. I was on the other side now. I could say that I had been accepted to those with the same fortune and could encourage those still waiting to hear. "It's just a matter of time," I said. I knew this was the right thing to say, even though I believed many of these people would never get a chance to hug their mailman.

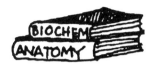

5. Medical School

THE CELEBRATION of my acceptance began to wear off as medical school grew near. The relaxation I had experienced became overshadowed by the fear that I needed better study habits to handle those famously tough medical school courses. When I went to college, I was told I had to compete against my peers in the upper ten percent of high schools across the nation. Now I would be in an even more elite group.

My medical school class was made up of one hundred future doctors. Most of their grade point averages were between 3.7 and 4.0. My grade point average was a 3.3, at best. Also, we had over thirty percent women, a record in the United States for that year.

I was happy. I had gotten into medical school and you either passed or failed. There were no more grades. The mail I received over the next three months started the experience. It informed me of the tuition, the price of my books, and the classes I would be taking the first year. Going to a state school saved an enormous amount of money. The tuition was only $250 a quarter, about one-fourth the cost of a private school.

Books were another story entirely. They weighed about ten pounds each and were so big that two could hardly fit into a book bag. Each book cost over $50 and I knew that when the class was over they would be of no use to me whatsoever. We were expected to buy them new but I immediately embarked on a mission to contact second-, third-, and fourth-year medical students to see if they would sell me their used books. Unbelievably, some of the students wanted to keep their books. They told me I could borrow the text and return it to them at the completion of the year. Such a deal. Especially the books where the important points had been highlighted in yellow.

I was amazed that anyone would consider keeping this oversized bundle of bullshit, but I was grateful and didn't ask any questions. Presumably some of them wanted to go into research and might need future references in this torture. Others felt as though their knowledge of medicine would be reflected by the stack of books on their shelves. Some doctors, I would find out, had the same kind of reasoning with diplomas. They put as many as possible on the wall to impress their patients. I always hung my diplomas on the wall directly over a garbage can. If they fell, their final resting place was appropriate.

Finally classes were announced. I would start with such notables as biochemistry, anatomy, physiology, and physical diagnosis. Biochemistry was, without a doubt, the most incredible pile of nonsense known to man. The entire time was spent memorizing chemical cycles that were forgotten within minutes after the exam. They had to be. Only two to three of these schemes could fit into the largest of brains.

The courses were taught by social misfits. You know, the ones with the outstanding personalities. They always showed up five minutes before class puffing on their pipes, testing the slide projector, and setting their timers for exactly fifty minutes of pure verbal diarrhea. When the clock struck 8:00 a.m. they didn't bother to say, "Good morning, class," but rather, "May I have the first slide, please." You sure may, straight up your tochis.

The name of the game was copy as fast as you could and don't worry about understanding the material. Oh, and occasionally, if you didn't understand something, you could go to their laboratories and ask the professors. Questions during class were discouraged and might make you look stupid in front of the other students. It was a challenge trying to find these professors in their laboratories between all of the test tubes, Bunsen burners, and beakers. Their answers echoed off containers steaming with hydrochloric acid.

Ph.D's are not real doctors. They are lab rats who would be lost outside the maze of the university. The game of assistant versus associate versus full professors is one of the most inept, political, and senseless debacles known to mankind. If they publish papers, they climb the proverbial ladder, even if they can't teach worth a damn. Tenured professors usually teach a few classes a year and make between $80,000 and $100,000 annually. They sit in their huge offices making irrelevant long distance phone calls at taxpayers' expense and writing papers that less than one out of a million people understand.

I don't mean to say there were no good professors. There were three. One went home to Portugal after my second year because he got screwed by a dean at the medical school. The second left because he didn't publish enough papers. He had been too busy being a good teacher. The third got a better offer from another college where he would be appreciated.

Anatomy was the best course of the first year. We went to the lab wearing white coats, like doctors, and dissected human cadavers. At least this had some relevance to medicine. As we dissected different parts of the body, we remembered. We learned.

The only problem with this class was that for three months your hands smelled like Formalin. This made it hard because when you picked your nose, you got high. When you hugged your girlfriend, she retreated. When you went to a restaurant, people politely asked the waiter if something was wrong in the kitchen. It didn't come off easily either. You could scrub your hands for hours. The smell persisted.

Occasionally it did come in handy. One Thanksgiving I returned to my parents' home for the traditional turkey dinner. I was upset when I was seated next to Kenny, an eight-year-old brat. So I simply put my arm around Kenny, making sure my smelly fingers settled close to his nose. He soon insisted he had an upset stomach from a "weird smell" and needed to go to the living room to lie down on the couch. Mission accomplished.

Physical diagnosis class was an attempt to make us feel like real doctors interviewing real patients. What we didn't know was that these patients were professionals, paid by the medical school to have first-year medical students interview them. We were then critiqued by one of the professors, who were doctors in private practice, not busy enough to practice full-time medicine. The school in return gave each of them the title of Clinical Professor. Whoop-de-doo.

These patients were great and usually very helpful, especially if the professors were late. This enabled us to interview them alone. I remember my patient who supposedly had a heart problem. I took his history. At this point, I knew very little about the heart, actually not much more than I know now. I remembered to ask open-ended questions like, "Can you tell me a little bit about your problem, Mr. Stark?" The patient answered that he had had chest pain for three years. He frequently had shortness of breath, medications weren't helping, and he was constantly tired. I told him it was too bad but he looked better now and wished him good luck.

As I got up to see how my friends were doing he said, "Don't you want to know about my smoking history?"

"Oh, certainly, I forgot to ask," I joked.

He explained, "I've smoked three packs a day for thirty years."

I told him that was the acid test for survival and he passed, so I offered to wait for my professor while he went out for a cigarette.

"But don't you want to know about my family history of heart disease?" he continued.

"I suppose so," I said.

"Three of my brothers died of heart attacks by the age of fifty and one sister had undergone open heart surgery at the age of forty-six," he stated.

I said, "At sixty-seven you have broken the odds and should live a long life. Mazel Tov."

After another hour, he told me all of the answers I needed for this same professor who had critiqued another student with him last week.

Typically, the professor showed up forty-five minutes late. When I explained that I had gone ahead and taken the patient's history, the professor agreed that this nice man could be excused. The professor then sat and discussed what I had done. Of course I looked like a star thanks to the patient. The professor said I had taken one of the best histories he could remember and begged me to consider a career in cardiology.

Most classes over the next two years were like the beer commercial, they just didn't get any better than this. It was hour after hour of memorizing facts that had no relevance to the clinical practice of medicine. I attended less than half of my classes. I didn't goof off.

Instead, I went to the library to memorize the notes that had been passed out in a syllabus prior to the lecture. This saved me several hours of sitting in a boring class each week. I needed the time to memorize all that trash.

Some of our teachers were uncommon human beings. One lanky physiology teacher slithered into class like a worm. His first lecture began with a statement of how useful his material would be and how we should pay careful attention. We had heard that line before. As he began lecturing, he suddenly stopped and addressed a girl in the front row who was knitting. "Excuse me, Miss, but I don't allow knitting while I'm lecturing," he said. The classroom was stunned.

I was afraid she would cry, but she rose to the occasion. She answered apologetically, "My roommate took this course last year and told me to bring my knitting to your lectures so I could stay awake." His face turned red. He continued lecturing. She continued knitting.

Another professor of otorhinolaryngology came to class only to notice that most of the students were seated in the back of the room. Very few people occupied the first two rows. This was standard so that if the material or the speaker were so dreadful it could not be tolerated, we could exit without much notice. "I'm depressed by what I see here class. My experience with students has proven that those of you who sit in the first row make first-rate doctors. Students who sit in the second row make second-rate doctors," he stated. I was in the ninth row which I calculated would be perfect for my interest in his subject matter.

The first two years were like treading water. Nothing else. There was no attempt to teach us anything that would be relevant to the rest of our careers. What I recall from my first two years could be stored in a thimble. Our professors constantly argued that this was not true and we would recall much more than we thought. This was just a ridiculous attempt to justify their presence.

The last two years of medical school were different. We trained at a large county hospital seeing real patients. Most importantly, we had more responsibility. In the third year, we were asked to prioritize our schedules. The choices were medicine, surgery, psychiatry, and pediatrics.

If you were so strung out by the first two years of studying that you needed some time off, a vacation if you will, you chose psychiatry. On this rotation nobody knew who you were or where you were supposed to be. But that was psychiatry. There were patient interviews we had to conduct through two-way mirrors, and some reading to be done, but that was it.

One interesting project had to be accomplished in psychiatry. A lengthy paper had to be written. I did mine on M.D. suicide. I was intrigued that the most common physician to commit suicide was a psychiatrist. So I read several articles on the subject and interviewed psychiatrists and some real doctors about the problem. I wanted to understand the rationale for this disease. The responses were fascinating. Some of the better answers were that doctors were under so much stress that they couldn't cope and just took the easy way out. They killed themselves. But this bothered me because it seemed it would take a lot of guts to kill yourself and most of the doctors I knew were jellyfish.

Another reason given was that physicians frequently became emotionally and sexually involved with their patients and when the facts were revealed, it caused divorces, violence, and subsequent deaths. Many of the physicians I knew were physically and emotionally undesirable. How could patients be attracted to them? Was it because they had money? All of the doctors I knew were so cheap that they wouldn't spend it on their lovers or even pay for a hotel room. They'd use either their offices or the back seat of a car.

What is my opinion? Doctors are among the strangest, most insecure people I know. They can't deal with their inadequacies and since they have an easy way to kill themselves, namely drugs, they do it. No muss, no fuss. It's not bloody and even better, it's not expensive. They don't have to pay for the drugs. They get them free from pharmaceutical representatives for "office use."

Psychiatrists are the nuttiest of all. They go into psychiatry to try to understand their own problems. Most of them fail. Let's face it. How many shrinks do you know that seem normal?

Just for fun, try to contact one in a pinch. All of them have answering machines. None of them have secretaries. The standard recording says, "Hello, this is Dr. Wanderer. I'm not available now, but if you would like to leave a message, please wait until the sound of the tone. Thank you."

I recently had a patient in the hospital who wanted to talk to one of these jokers. I made five calls and left a message on all of their machines. The first one called me back in three hours, two called back within five hours, and the other two the following day. I was glad my patient wasn't going crazy.

My psychiatry rotation was finally over. If you didn't have the ability to communicate with your patients by the time you entered medical school, this rotation couldn't help you. We all agreed that understanding patients and their problems was vital, but this rotation was for the birds.

I chose pediatrics next. I wanted to get this rotation out of the way so I could begin to concentrate on medicine and surgery. However, pediatrics was clinical. I needed to learn about medications and their effects but I couldn't pay too much attention to the doses because they would be inadequate for adults, except midgets.

Again we worked in the county hospital and clinic. The method of learning was always the same. As the student, I saw the patient first, did a history and physical examination, and took my report to the fourth-year student. Together we returned to the patient, where the fourth-year student said, "Dr. Mays tells me you've had an earache for three days and it's not getting better." The patient was examined again by my superior. Together we descended upon the intern, the real M.D., and reported the problem.

He would say, "It sounds like otitis media (an ear infection) and I agree with you that a three-day course of antibiotics is appropriate." I spent six weeks listening to babies cry, looking in hundreds of ears, cleaning out buckets of wax, and avoiding overreactive mothers.

Pediatric rounds on the hospital wards were unbelievably boring. Here I was exposed to what the third-year students called "pimping." This was when professors tried to make you look bad by asking difficult questions. Even if you got the answer right, they found some piece of information that you had left out.

This was good for people who loved to read pediatric journals. "Who can tell me the incidence of influenza in children under the age of four in Malaysia?" the professor asked. Who could care? When none of us knew, we were told to go and read the latest pediatric journal as we would be quizzed on it tomorrow.

I hated pediatrics because I love happy, healthy children. I felt sad when I saw them gravely ill in the pediatric intensive care unit, hooked up to six monitors and breathing through a tube. Kids are supposed to be healthy, resistant to almost anything.

This was clearly not my bag and I knew it. But I got through it. I saw virtually no pediatric orthopedics on this rotation, which made me even less interested.

There was one incident on my pediatric rotation that I will never forget. It happened one night when I was on call. Don't think being on call was a real privilege. I stayed in the hospital all night. The rooms were quite luxurious, complete with a sink and a cot. The floor plan was similar to prison, but the prisoners didn't take night calls. When my senior house staff officer got a call, I went too. I followed like a dog.

One night I was awakened by a call from my intern who said she had to go over to the clinic to see a baby with a fever. I looked at my watch. It was 3:30 a.m. I quickly jumped into my clothes from yesterday and hustled after her. I was so tired, I didn't even brush my teeth. We entered the exam room together to see the patient, as the usual protocol used during the day took too long. We just wanted to see the patient and get back to sleep.

An indigent mother was holding an eight-month-old baby who was sound asleep. She explained that the child had been irritable over the past week and she was wondering if the child had an ear infection. Admittedly, the child had improved over the past few days. She said, "The main reason I came tonight was that I knew you wouldn't be busy and I wouldn't have to wait to be seen." My usually calm intern turned red with anger, but kept amazingly cool as she explained we only saw emergencies at night and that the woman would have to call for an appointment in the daytime clinic.

This is why I believe in capital punishment. This was a crime. This was a total misuse of our time and the system. I was tired and irritable, so I got her name. Justice had to be served, and I knew my intern was too nice to take action.

When I arrived at the clinic the next morning, I checked over the list to see if the woman had called in. She had. I was on a mission. I continually checked the clinic waiting room and when she finally showed up, I deviously kept putting her chart under a couple of others so she would have to wait. Luckily the baby slept soundly in her arms. I didn't want the baby to be penalized. I was so pleased when she was seen at 4:15 p.m. for her 1:30 p.m. appointment. Another doctor found the examination to be normal. On the way out, the mother said to me, "Didn't I see you here in the clinic last night?" I responded that she must be mistaken as I had just gotten off my psychiatry rotation.

Now that I was finished with the two obligatory rotations of my third year, I was ready to start medical school. I decided there wasn't much reason to start surgery without some knowledge of medical problems and specific medications, so I decided to do my medicine rotation next.

This was the most incredible exercise in one-upmanship I had ever seen. Who had read the most journals? Who could quote the last ten years of the *New England Journal of Medicine*? I was really a fish out of water because I hated reading medical journals.

The medicine rotation began with the intern handing me a list of four patients. I was supposed to study their charts, then ask questions about the patients and their conditions the following morning. You must understand that each of the medical patients in a county hospital had at least ten different problems documented in eight volumes of charts. Each chart was two inches thick.

The diseases common to all patients on the medical ward of a county hospital included chronic liver disease, pancreatitis, and organic brain syndrome. This was because they all drank like sieves and many were chronic alcoholics. Most of them were in congestive heart failure and their electrolyte balance was so far out of whack because their kidney cells were drunk. And, of course, all of these problems were interrelated. The first night I spent three hours going through volumes of charts. This was their monthly visit.

I was determined to make a good start now that I was finally getting down to what I needed to know. Though I had no intention of being an internist, I wanted to make a good impression my first day on rounds.

I started off less than impressive. My first professor was a woman. Well, sort of. She weighed 250 pounds and stood six feet three inches tall. She scared the shit out of me. She treated us all the same, like total incompetents.

"Dr. Mays, tell me all you know about the electrolyte imbalances seen in patients with chronic renal failure," she barked. She actually called on me. Who in the hell did she think she was? But I had studied and I knew it. I was petrified as I answered correctly. I could tell she was annoyed that I knew the answer. She countered by saying my answer was partially accurate but incomplete. I felt like saying I wanted a second opinion. The entire three months was like this. But you learned by this technique—fright.

After you saw enough patients with these types of problems, you learned about kidneys and livers. Rounds became so boring they were painful, but I had to do it. Fortunately, many of the professors thought the students were a nuisance, so they paid no attention to us on rounds. Our questions were considered unintelligent and we were told to go over them with the house staff after rounds.

One of the things I liked about medicine was that I was allowed to do procedures. I got to draw all the blood I could handle, as I was better with my hands than with my brain. This was why I wanted to be a surgeon. I was called upon frequently and became the designated errand boy. "Hey Dr. Mays, run down and draw a quick blood sample from Mrs. Robles before rounds because Dr. Frederick will want to have an updated blood count on her leukemia status," my intern dictated. What was really stupid was that the last blood sample was drawn four hours earlier and it would have been much less expensive and traumatic to the patient if we had just made up a number. The professor would have never known the difference.

There were other great procedures too. I became very proficient at inserting subclavian intravenous lines into the large veins draining into the heart. These were used often in emergency room patients needing large quantities of fluids in a hurry, like patients with bullet wounds.

One day an intern told me there was a very sick old man with liver disease in the intensive care unit. He had too much fluid in his belly, which was impairing his breathing. This intern knew I was good with the needle and, since I had seen him do this procedure once before, he asked me if I was comfortable taking off more abdominal fluid. Of course I was.

I got my tools, numbed the skin where I was to insert the large needle, and easily withdrew a couple thousand cc's without any difficulty. The next morning the intern told me I probably took off a little too much fluid because the patient went into cardiac arrest due to electrolyte imbalance and died. But the intern admitted that the belly definitely looked better.

Another procedure I liked was bone marrow aspiration. This was usually done in the hip bone when we needed to look at blood cells in people with blood disorders such as leukemia. I was introduced to this procedure by a professor of hematology who tried to demonstrate the technique on the breastbone of a patient. This particular bone was so brittle and soft that the professor went right through the breastbone, into the heart, and the patient nearly bled to death in front of my eyes. This made me uncomfortable with the breastbone technique.

Emergency call on medicine was every third night. This was torture. I was often up the entire night, got no sleep, and hated the patients. None of them were young, none of them were in good shape, none of them got significantly better, and most of them looked like hell. I like making people well, getting them back on the field.

I saved the best for last—surgery. I started on general surgery because I had to learn how to tie knots and take care of the typical problems frequently encountered with all surgical patients, like wound care, fluid replacement, and general techniques.

The service was headed by Dr. Mummy, the chief of surgery. He was a crony of the dean and was brought to the university for political reasons. Dr. Mummy didn't know anything about taking care of patients or surgical techniques. He looked like a corpse, smoked a pipe, and always sat in the front row at grand rounds so he could question the residents giving the presentations.

Grand rounds was a choice event. Once a week, students and surgical specialists, including private practice physicians, filled an auditorium. As students, we presented our care of patients, which was then critiqued by the professors and local physicians. We knew it was imperative to be polite and responsive to their suggestions and comments, as our surgical programs were dependent upon the participation of these local physicians for accreditation purposes. The beat goes on.

I remember one private doc saying, "This is similar to the lady I saw last week in my office. Her presenting symptoms were the same and her laboratory values were similar. I performed an immediate cholecystectomy and she went home three days later." But everyone knew most of these guys were full of it and probably never in their lives had seen a patient like we were discussing. They merely wanted to stand up and tell everyone how smart they were. At the end of the conferences, Dr. Mummy would summarize, "This has been one of the best grand rounds I can remember." The trouble was he couldn't recall he had made that same statement the last four weeks in a row.

General surgery was boring. These guys loved opening up the belly, putting their oversized paws into the abdominal cavity, and feeling around. "The bowel feels entirely normal. The liver and spleen are normal in size and shape. The gallbladder is in the correct position, and I don't feel any stones. The pancreas is normal through-out its entirety," was the standard jargon. I always wondered what the hell they were doing in the belly if all of these things were normal.

Next I moved on to urology. I called it the stream team. I enjoyed this because I was with a resident who liked to teach and who let me operate. The resident looked like a moon man. He had a narrow face, little hair, thick, rectangular-shaped glasses, and a small mustache. He let me close wounds, tie knots, and insert catheters, so I felt like I was needed and appreciated.

It was on this service that I met the biggest asshole surgeon I would ever meet. He was a six-foot-four-inches-tall professor with a malignant personality and a big mustache. He had the worst temper I had ever seen.

I did a case with Dr. Handlebar and a resident. The resident unfor-tunately made a small mistake with a suture. Dr. Handlebar smacked his wrist with the suction instrument. The resident didn't say a word. I was so angry I wanted to retaliate, but I was just a lowly student.

Later in the case, the scrub nurse didn't have the special tool that Dr. Handlebar wanted, so she handed him something similar, hoping it would take its place. He turned away from the table. With all his might, he threw it against the wall. The scrub nurse began to cry. The next day she turned in her resignation, but was talked into stay-ing if it were written in her contract that she never had to work with this tyrant again.

The third year was almost history. I saved what I had hoped would be the best for last—orthopedic surgery. This was my baby. This was what I wanted to do. This was what I wanted to be—a bone setter. I had several goals in mind. I wanted to learn about this department and whether it would be a worthwhile program for my residency training. Secondly, I wanted to get to know the faculty to see if I wanted to learn my life's work from them. Finally, I wanted to see what type of orthopedics they did. Was it mostly trauma, reconstructive surgery, total joint replacement, hand surgery, or what?

As with most county hospitals, there was an enormous amount of trauma. We took care of all the solid citizens—drunks and motorcycle riders. In addition, there was a fair amount of other disciplines, including hand surgery, total joint replacement, and spine surgery. I felt the faculty members all had very different personalities and varying degrees of competency.

The best part of the program was the chairman, Dr. Buttons. He was an elderly gentleman who came from an esteemed midwestern clinic. He was soft-spoken and a true gentleman. He was not interested in making the residents or students look bad but rather in making his program look good. He forever emphasized certain points of the program: the year-end exam scores of the residents, the evaluations of the students, and the ability of the residents to graduate and pass the National Orthopedic Board Examination.

The rest of the faculty was less impressive. The head of the total joint rotation, Dr. Smooth, was an egotistical maniac who thought he was a sex symbol. His main ambition in life was to be the chief of a residency program, and he was only hanging around until the appropriate opportunity surfaced.

Another member of the faculty was a very capable Japanese man, Dr. Nadaworda. He was nice, but couldn't speak English well. I could never understand him, nor could anyone else.

Dr. Pipe, the chief of the hand service, was pleasant but a terror in surgery. He frequently lost his cool and yelled at everyone. He was another one just biding time until a better position surfaced. He wasn't going to get tenure at this university because he seldom published a scientific paper. Not only that, he wasn't a good teacher. But he was friendly with Dr. Smooth, so when a chairmanship opened up for Dr. Smooth, I felt sure they would both be gone.

The other full-time professor, Dr. Drill, was a mechanical nightmare. He was pleasant and friendly toward students, but I doubted I could train under him. The residents told me he was a horrible technician. They had a standing joke that he loved to fix things. As soon as a resident began a surgical case with Dr. Drill, he or she would deliberately break an instrument so that Dr. Drill would retreat to the back table and fix it as the resident quickly finished the surgery.

Dr. Spud was the head of the scoliosis and spine service. He was interested in something very few orthopedic surgeons wanted to be involved in, taking care of children with severe spinal deformities. He was a peaceful man who devoted some time to the students, but not a great deal. He was nice to his patients. I liked this because these patients and families went through great emotional trauma both before and after these horrendous, highly complicated surgical procedures. This guy was clearly the best in our area and I respected him for that. It was a part of orthopedics I wasn't terribly interested in, but I knew I had to know something about it in the long run.

My conclusions after being on the service were that this program was weak in teaching experience, but certainly adequate if no one else wanted me. I enjoyed most of the residents in orthopedic surgery, and they were willing to help teach students. This was especially true for me since I showed an interest in orthopedics. They even let me do some surgery and that was exciting. I got to set a lot of fractures in the emergency room and I became very proficient at casting and splinting. I did more reading than in all of my first two years in medical school because I was doing something I liked. I was stimulated. I found if I just picked out three or four subjects a night and read about them, I learned a lot and I reassured myself that this was the right field for me.

I was also interested in the involvement of the orthopedic surgeons in the community. This program relied heavily on their participation and residents were frequently farmed out to the community hospitals for three-month rotations with a private guy. There were several docs who participated heavily.

One was a big, fat Army doctor, Dr. Round, who was interested in orthopedic pathology. There were about five people in the whole country who were interested in this subject. It was embarrassing when he lectured to the students on orthopedic tumors because the snoring was so loud, you couldn't hear the lecture. The residents joked that they wore cervical collars to cut down on the neck sprains that occurred while nodding off during his boring lectures. But his information on orthopedic tumors was necessary for the Board exams. He was a good sport, though. He knew it was the end of the day and everyone was tired. He was also a decent clinician and had several helpful hints about the practice of general office orthopedics.

Then there was Dr. Mac, the chief of the local prepaid health plan, the Free for All Clinic. He was another nice guy, but boring. If you asked him the time, he gave you a full explanation on how to build a watch. He loved quizzing the students. If you could stand this, he contributed some good information and also had a fair understanding of children's orthopedics.

My rotation on orthopedics was definitely worthwhile, not only because I learned about the faculty, but because they learned about me too. I felt it was paramount that I be well liked or I had no chance of getting into the residency program.

The final year of school was completely elective and I could choose my classes and experiences. There was an interesting thought process that went through my head about this upcoming year. I had had it up to my cervical spine with being a student. I wanted to start having more responsibilities and I was determined that all of my electives allow me this. I might have longer hours and more stress than many fourth-year students wanting to take it easy, but I needed to be "in the barrel." I wanted to be on the front line and learn how to be a doctor firsthand. I wanted to accomplish in my fourth year what an intern essentially accomplished, thus saving a year. If I could go through this grueling acting internship my fourth year in school, maybe I wouldn't have to be an intern when I graduated from medical school.

An exceptional student could graduate from medical school and go straight into an orthopedic residency without an internship if he or she demonstrated an unusually high aptitude. There were only a few programs like this in the country. Aggie University had one of them. I knew it would take some luck, but why not try? Crazier things had happened. Remember, I got into medical school.

I arranged for some intensive medical and surgical acting internships where I would get good practical experience as a student. In addition, I had to start applying for orthopedic residencies. The residents and faculty members helped me find the programs with the best reputations.

In between these tough fourth-year acting internships, I took time out to visit residency programs for more, you guessed it, personal interviews. Acceptance into residency programs was more dependent upon politics and recommendations than upon grades or exam scores. Fortunately, many of the orthopedic faculty liked me well enough to highly recommend me.

I went on one interview back East and they did things a little differently than I had been used to during my medical school interviews. This particular orthopedic department had several faculty members interview me. They allowed me to carry my confidential folder from one interviewer to the next. After my second interview, I had the incredible desire to find out what these professors back home actually had to say about me. But where could I go? Is this honest? Damned straight. I found a men's room, equipped with a stall. I opened my folder and began to read. I studied the file closely. I had no interruptions, thank God. I would have lost my cool and probably any chance of a spot there if I had been caught. You know what? I was pleased. People really had nice things to say about me. Even some professors from my first two years. I was amazed. I was complimented. I headed for my next interview, mission accomplished.

This final year was really exciting. I traveled to prospective residencies and worked around the state on acting internships. I worked long hours, frequently in frustration, but I learned a lot about medicine and, more importantly, about how to take care of sick patients. I started to feel I could manage a very sick patient, even one who was dying, all by myself. I knew how to handle insulin needs of diabetics, irregular beats of heart patients, and what to do when patients stopped breathing. I was finally feeling like a doctor of medicine. This was what it was all about. Even though treating very sick patients wasn't my long-term goal, I felt good about myself and what I knew.

I was frequently humbled, as there was always someone around who knew more than I did. But I learned to live with this, even though at times it was humiliating. It was all part of the game. I was never a scholar, so I learned to accept early on that everyone was scholastically smarter than I. I was destined to be a good clinician and a quality orthopedic surgeon. I took good care of my patients. This I felt was numero uno. This was my belief in medicine. Take good care of your patients and they will take good care of you.

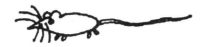

6. Fourth-Year Rat Surgery

I HAD always been enthusiastic about human anatomy. I liked studying muscles and bones. I decided it would be a real feather in my cap to boast a master's degree in human anatomy on my applications for an orthopedic residency. I wanted to look as good as possible so I could avoid an internship and go directly from medical school to a residency program. It wasn't that much extra work, only a few extra classes while completing my fourth year of medical school. I would have to complete a small project and pass an oral examination. All of this could be done before I graduated.

I got some great teaching experience. It was customary for human anatomy graduate students to teach laboratory classes for the pre-nursing and pre–physical therapy students. If you ever want to learn a subject backwards and forwards, teach it. During the first session, I was asked several questions I could not answer. I began studying diligently before the classes. I couldn't have the teacher knowing less than the student.

I loved it because anatomy was something I liked and I wanted to remember. The students liked it too. They loved the dissections which I had completed and labeled on my own time. They said it was fun to identify the tags on the models and specimens, and it had been fun for me to prepare them. It was not something irrelevant and useless like setting up an integral in calculus or memorizing a biochemistry cycle. What I did not anticipate, however, was that this would be the start of a long love relationship with teaching, not to mention other lifelong relationships; one of the prenursing students later became my wife.

The professor who supervised the teaching assistants called me in at the end of the semester, as was customary, to comment on my teaching evaluations. I thought I had done a good job, but you never know. She stated my evaluations were among the most impressive she had ever seen and this would go a long way in helping me achieve my master's degree in human anatomy. I was pleased.

There was one more major hurdle in the degree, however. I needed a project that dealt with something experimental or research-oriented. I was committed to finding something relevant, something that would help me in my career as a surgeon. I had heard that Dr. Pipe, the hand surgeon in the medical school's orthopedic department, was experimenting with microvascular surgical techniques. He was trying to perfect methods for sewing tiny blood vessels which would then reestablish blood flow to digits like fingers or toes. He used rat tails to practice his surgical skills. The artery that goes down the middle of the rat tail is approximately the same size as the blood vessel running down the side of your finger.

Dr. Pipe was a charming and handsome gentleman who smoked. The problem with this habit was that it created a major tremor in his hands, so he could not sew these minute vessels. He welcomed a young man with a steady hand to help him finish the project.

I had to get the rats from the veterinary school and put them to sleep with a liquid anesthetic. After a minimal sterile preparation, I would cut open the tail, dissect out the artery, cut it, and reattach it with our surgical technique. The trick was to sew it back together well enough that in six weeks, when we shot dye into the rat's vascular system, the blood clearly flowed across the sutured area. This may sound simple, but considering that the vessel was about the size of a sharp pencil tip, the chance of establishing blood flow through it after being severed was not great.

After I practiced on three rats and got my technique down, I was ready. I should mention that this entire procedure had to be done under a very high-powered microscope and that the suture was so small and light that it floated in air. But this work actually came quite easy for me. I knew I couldn't be any worse than my mentor, who shook so badly I thought he was doing the boogaloo.

The hardest part of the case for me was anesthetizing the rat. Oh I'm not talking about putting an innocent animal to sleep. Getting him to stay still long enough to breathe the anesthetic was difficult. Sometimes the smell of the stuff in the room made me feel a little high. But it relaxed my hands, which made for a more successful experiment.

The procedure took about an hour to perform and the rat usually awakened a few hours later. For two weeks, I inspected the wounds daily. Then at six weeks, I put them back to sleep and injected dye to see if the operated vessel was patent (open). I recorded my results on twenty rats. Over eighty-five percent worked. Our technique was successful.

Even better, my results looked so good that I actually published a paper. Responses to the publication were favorable. Imagine me, publishing. Maybe I could be a professor and get tenure. Maybe I could become a member of the Flying Aggies and swing down to the Almond Patch for lunch every day at the university's expense.

The remainder of my master's work was done between electives and acting internships my fourth year. The light was now visible. Could I accomplish the "big three"? Graduate from medical school, get a master's degree in human anatomy, and be accepted into an orthopedic residency directly out of medical school? At least now I knew I could accomplish two of the three.

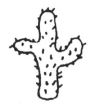

7. The Great Phoenix

DURING my fourth and final year of medical school, in addition to completing some important acting internships, I felt the need to find a good solid stint in orthopedic surgery where I would have some serious responsibility. That way, if I could slide into an orthopedic surgery residency right out of medical school, I would be one step ahead of the rest of the clan. But where could I find such an experience on short notice?

I happened to meet a hardworking intern at the hospital one day. He wore the usual dirty, waist-high white lab coat with a stethoscope, reflex hammer, and three syringes sticking out of one pocket. In the other pocket he had a medical manual, four meal tickets, and an ophthalmoscope to peer into eyeballs. He and I hit it off well. He had an interest in orthopedic surgery but wanted to do an internship in medicine first. He was not as sold on orthopedics as I was but he did have some good advice.

He had recently worked at a county hospital in Arizona as an extern in orthopedic surgery. He was the first student there to have ever done this. "Don't go unless you can endure some heavy emotional tension," he said. The head of the program had criticized him from the moment he stepped into the hospital and never said boo to him when he left. No "Nice having you here" or "Thanks for your interest in our program." But my friend admitted he did learn orthopedics. Every day he was in the emergency room, on the front line, doing orthopedic care.

This sounded like just what the doctor ordered. I figured if I could take such an unreasonable amount of flack from as many medical misfits as I had thus far, certainly I was up to the task of handling this kingpin. I wrote another one of my patronizing, humble letters about how I had heard that this was one of the best acting (on-the-job) externships in orthopedic surgery and was there a chance I could be blessed with this outstanding experience? Once again, the old adage of "say what they want to hear" came through. I was accepted in the late winter.

The timing was perfect because it allowed me to first complete some good medical training to handle very sick patients. Even better, the rotation in Arizona was close to the end of the year, so I wouldn't forget how to set bones when I got to my residency.

As I prepared to go off to the desert, I took the time to make an appointment with the chairman of the orthopedic department at Aggie University Medical School.

Oh, I forgot. Nowadays you can't say chairman. You have to say chair. Nonsense. You sit in a chair.

Where was I anyway? Oh, the reason I made the appointment was to once again appear humble and let the hierarchy know I was still very interested in their orthopedic residency program.

I also wanted to get Dr. Buttons's opinion on other programs now that I had some expertise in microvascular surgery. He felt that the best residency in the country was in North Carolina. The internationally known chairman of the department was recognized for his outstanding achievements in microvascular surgery.

Was this another case of being in the right place at the right time? My chairman and this noted hand surgeon were going to be together on a panel the following week in Chicago, and Dr. Buttons asked if I wanted him to question this famed professor about possible residency slots. It certainly sounded like a good idea. After all, I knew where Dr. Buttons was coming from. He was thinking that if one of his students was accepted into the most renowned orthopedic program in the country, it would be a feather in his cap and would make the university look good.

I had heard in many circles that this program was one of the better ones in the country and I knew Dr. Buttons was being honest. But wait a minute. Why should I want to go there? I could think of several reasons not to, one being that I would have to go to North Carolina. Second, it was a five-year program and I was still working toward getting through an orthopedic surgery residency in four years. Third, the program was very academically oriented and I was about as interested in academics as I was in chimney sweeping. Fourth, the program emphasized hand surgery and I wasn't interested in being a hand surgeon. I only did the rat research experiments to develop my surgical skills, especially with fine objects. Finally, I had heard that this esteemed chairman was hard-driving and not much fun. But, in any event, I seemed to have several possibilities as the fourth year continued to roll on.

It wouldn't be long before I would have to declare my choices for the so-called matching program. This was a system whereby a medical student wrote down his choices of internships or residencies in the order of his preference. At the same time, each program prioritized its choices of students and the two systems were "matched." It was a national attempt to put interns and residents where the students wanted to go, assuming the institution wanted them. It really makes sense now that I think about it. However, at the time I was filling out all the papers, it seemed ridiculously cumbersome and complicated.

There was one problem. The matching program only applied to the usual postmedical training programs like internships and established five-year orthopedic residencies. There was no match for the programs I needed to become a first-year orthopedic resident immediately out of medical school. I was not foolish enough to forget that I might not make it into one of these special programs and therefore I was obligated to go through the match.

But before I filled out my final choices, I had some large decisions to make. Which schools should I list first? What was going to happen with North Carolina? The Arizona opportunity sounded outstanding, but I had not been there yet.

When Dr. Buttons returned from his meeting in Chicago, we chatted about his conversation with the Southern professor. If I went to North Carolina for an interview and was well received, there was a good chance that I would be offered a position. The professor had reminded Dr. Buttons that he took only the cream of the crop. There was no way of guaranteeing my acceptance. Should I fly all the way to North Carolina, just in case? I was hesitant to spend that kind of time and money.

Dr. Buttons suggested I call the chairman himself and the two of us could have a man-to-man conversation. Was there any way he would be willing to accept me into the program without an interview? I knew I was dreaming, but what the hell. He returned my call late the next night at home. I trembled when I heard he was on the phone — the big cheese himself.

I started with the usual. "Thank you so much for returning my call and taking the time out of your busy schedule," I said. "Dr. Buttons told me what a wonderful man you are and I truly enjoyed reading all of your publications in the orthopedic literature." Have you had enough? Wait, there's more. I explained to him that I had this incredible desire to work with the most famous hand surgeon in the world and I believed my specialized training in microvascular surgery further qualified me for the program. I continued, "My problem, Professor, is that I'm leaving soon for an orthopedic rotation in Arizona and I don't have time to come for an interview. In addition, I've been working so hard on my studies, I haven't earned any money to finance the trip."

I found out why his personality was considered rigid. He explained he had never accepted an orthopedic resident into his program without a personal interview. Being accepted without going back East was out of the question. I asked if there might be an alumnus in our area who could interview me, but he said that was "hogwash." He had no confidence in what other people thought about his prospective residents. He did say that from all he had heard about me, I stood a decent chance of acceptance. He added that the only other resident in his program with a specific interest in microvascular surgery was graduating this year. The situation was potentially perfect for me to carry on much of his ongoing research. I again thanked him for returning my call, and he reiterated that I should schedule the interview with his secretary.

I spoke with Dr. Buttons, who suggested I go for the interview, but I procrastinated because I didn't want to go. And I didn't.

My problem still existed. How should I list the programs on my match? Where would I list Arizona, even though I knew the least about this program and had not even visited the hospital? I hadn't stood before the program head who had frightened my friend. Somehow I had the best feeling about Arizona. The program was apparently very solid and without the usual amount of academic crap that muddied most university programs. So that was it. I decided to put Arizona first, Aggie University second, and North Carolina third. I mailed off the match, packed my bags, and headed for the desert.

My wife and I found a small apartment near the hospital. She was a good sport about the move and volunteered to work through the local nursing registry to pay for our expenses. Since I would be gone most days and many nights, she could work many shifts.

The first day I met with Dr. Flaps. He was a noble-looking man with almost no hair. He was very matter-of-fact and looked at me over the top of his glasses. He explained my schedule, said I was there by choice, and if I applied myself, I would leave with a tremendous wealth of knowledge. I was excited. This was what I wanted to hear.

He sent me off to meet the residents in the orthopedic clinic of this large county hospital. They were nice, but the overwhelming feeling I got was that they were burned out from the huge amount of patients and surgery. If after a few days of orientation I wanted to be first on call in the emergency room at night, it was mine for the asking.

For the next few days, I familiarized myself with the system. I made rounds early in the morning with the residents and the "main man" himself, Dr. Flaps. He really wasn't bad at all. He was stern with the residents but fair. He criticized their traction setups on the beds, but from what I'd seen on my orthopedic rotation at Aggie University, they needed criticism. He questioned their surgical indications in the clinic but seemed to have valid suggestions.

The real eye-opener was the fracture clinic after rounds each day. Every morning we went over all the fractures seen the night before in the emergency room. Each case, big or small, was presented to Dr. Flaps. He reviewed the fracture mechanism of injury (how the fracture occurred), the treatment, and the outcome with the resident who had handled the case. He was tough. I sat in horror when the resident mistakenly proposed the wrong mechanism of injury my first day and Dr. Flaps jumped all over him. When a fracture was set inappropriately, the resident was told to call the patient at home immediately and bring him back to set it correctly.

Did I really want to be on this chopping block? Yes. I was learning the stuff. It was trial by fire. Why was I there if I didn't want to learn? I sucked it up. I knew I would take a few lumps and bumps, but I would be well qualified in the fracture care of orthopedic patients after this ordeal.

I did take my lumps. I spent three straight nights in the emergency room to learn the ropes. I wanted the nurses to know who I was, and I wanted Dr. Flaps and the residents to know I was serious about being on my own. I hoped to gain some respect.

Then it happened. On the fourth day, one of the residents was sick and it was his night in the barrel. The chief resident told Dr. Flaps I was ready and I should get the nod. Dr. Flaps reluctantly agreed. I gratefully accepted the offer. I agreed to call him at home if I had any questions. He assured me he would arrive quickly if there were a serious problem or a life-threatening orthopedic emergency.

I called my wife to say my big opportunity had finally arrived. After all these years in training, I was going to get my first big chance to practice orthopedic surgery, even if it was without a license. I was being supervised from a distance. I was psyched. I invited her to have dinner with me in the hospital cafeteria. Now that I was the in-house orthopedic surgeon, I couldn't possibly leave.

Fortunately, my first showdown was relatively quiet. I saw four fractures and sewed up three deep lacerations. The fractures were familiar and I dealt with them appropriately. Between calls I spent time reading about their mechanism of injury and prognosis. Since I had been awakened only once during the night, I could face the firing squad in the morning looking fairly alert.

I got up early to make sure all the x-rays were in order for the fracture conference. I didn't want to look disorganized. Following rounds, we proceeded to the fracture clinic. I was petrified. Dr. Flaps was going to gun me down at the O.K. Corral.

The first lady I presented had an unstable finger fracture that I had reduced (pulled straight) and splinted. He said the alignment of the bone was adequate, but that the reduction would probably not hold and I would have to reset it in a few days. He said it was worth a try and to follow it closely by x-ray. He was impressed that I had already made a follow-up appointment for her tomorrow in case the fracture became crooked. He suggested that I probably had some "beginner's luck" and that the fracture would turn out fine.

The next man came in with a severely displaced wrist fracture. Dr. Flaps noticed that there were two reduction films which meant I had done it twice before I got it right. Again, when I presented the patient, I admitted I wasn't pleased with my initial reduction and wanted to try to make it better. He agreed that my first reduction was terrible but my second was better.

The other two cases were more standard, so he decided to challenge me on the mechanism of injuries and the long-term prognoses. But I was ready for the task. With the exception of a few thoughts, I seemed to hold my own. At the end there was no mention of a good job or a bad job. As we left the room, I felt no news was good news.

The Phoenix rotation clearly had more potential than I had expected. The residents turned out to be very overworked. They were either running to the operating room or hurrying to start a clinic. Because of this they gave me a lot of good bread-and-butter surgical cases and they were fair with me. If I saw a patient in the emergency room or clinic and worked them up properly, they let me take care of them, including doing the surgery if required. That seemed fair, you might say, but at many institutions after the student did all the preliminary work, the resident or intern stole the case. Not in Arizona.

As advertised, Dr. Flaps turned out to be different. He wasn't unpleasant, just unfriendly. He occasionally chatted with me about a patient who had a difficult problem. If he saw an interesting case in the clinic, he was very good about sharing it with me. But I couldn't read him. That was frustrating, because I liked his program, I liked Arizona, and I began to think I might want to train there.

Did he like me? Did he think I was any good? The only positives were that he seldom criticized me and often referred to my workups in discussions with patients. "I know you've been having trouble with your hip, Mrs. Mesa, and Dr. Mays explained to me about your previous injuries," he said. He knew my name and spent some time with me and this was a far cry from what my intern friend back home had described.

When I look back over my professional career, one of the most outstanding days occurred on unlucky Friday the thirteenth in Arizona.

I had four days left on my rotation. I was in the clinic writing in a chart when the head nurse told me I had received a call from Dr. Smooth at Aggie University. He had asked that I call him back as soon as possible. I had no idea what the call was about, but since he was not the program chairman, I doubted it had anything to do with the residency.

I was wrong. When I immediately returned his call, Dr. Smooth explained that the residency selection committee would very much like me to consider returning to Aggie University for my residency following an internship.

I paused a moment and said to myself, NO WAY. I explained to Dr. Smooth in my usual humble narrative that I was honored that the staff was interested in me, but that my interests in Aggie University revolved around the possibility that I would be taken right out of medical school without an internship. I further explained, "As you probably know (but just in case you don't), I've been doing acting internships in medicine all year long to avoid an internship and to better prepare myself for an immediate orthopedic residency. Furthermore, I've visited other orthopedic programs recently, and there are several places more suited to my specific needs for private practice." (So read between the lines, Dr. Smooth. If you folks want me badly enough, you'd best grab me now, right out of medical school.) I was hoping I didn't come across too abrasive. I hoped he wouldn't hang up on me.

I was depressed when he explained that the committee had already chosen the residents for next year. The die was cast. I was not one of them. I thanked him for his call and told him I would have to think about his generous offer. I promised to get back to him by the end of the week. I told him how much I was enjoying my rotation in Arizona and how fond I had grown of Dr. Flaps. I vividly recall Dr. Smooth joking and telling me he didn't want to come right out and beg me, but "you must know how much the faculty at Aggie University respects you." He was sure, after I had time to think, I would accept his offer.

That afternoon, between surgical cases, a rare opportunity arose when Dr. Flaps was sitting in the surgeons' lounge with the senior resident. I sat down, listened and laughed, especially when Dr. Flaps spoke. Then it happened. The senior resident was paged. When he left the room I bashfully told Dr. Flaps about the phone call from Dr. Smooth, and that I would welcome any advice concerning how a student interested in orthopedic surgery chooses a residency program.

I was concerned as he peered away from me. "I'm sorry to hear you're thinking of returning to California, because I was going to offer you a place here next year before you left on Friday," he stated. My heart started pounding. I quickly smiled to show him how much I appreciated his offer. He commented how all the residents had expressed confidence and happiness with my abilities and they all agreed I should be offered a position. I explained I was interested in a four-year program, which he did not offer, but if I weren't accepted into one of those programs, I would be ecstatic about choosing Arizona as my training ground. He told me to let him know as soon as possible. I was so thrilled. He actually talked to me. He actually looked me in the eye and told me he was happy with my performance.

That day a new pinnacle had been reached in my medical career. I was not only close to finishing medical school, but I had been offered two positions in orthopedic residency programs in the same day. Although I was feeling happy and a real sense of achievement, I still had not accomplished my big objective—a four-year program. But what the hell, you can't have everything.

After two more cases in surgery with Dr. Flaps and the senior resident, I asked a junior resident to cover for me so I could take my wife to dinner to celebrate my two offers. We laughed at the fact that Friday the thirteenth was not so unlucky. We discussed the two places which were very different.

Arizona was beautiful in the winter and filled with snowbirds. It was very hot in the summer, flat, and with little culture compared to home. But California was crowded and both sets of our parents lived there. We agreed it would be nice to get away from the families for awhile. After all, five years wasn't forever and we could tolerate anything for that length of time.

The remainder of the week was fun. Everyone, even Dr. Flaps, was especially nice to me in an effort to persuade me to return. Dr. Flaps even arranged to take me to lunch on my last day and I don't remember my predecessor having had that privilege. As a matter of fact, he told me that when he left, he didn't think anyone even knew he was gone. No one had said good-bye. I hadn't heard anything bad about him while I was there, but come to think of it, I hadn't heard anything about him at all.

As Friday dawned, I was a happy camper. I would be even happier as the day progressed. I brought cookies my wife had baked to Dr. Flaps's secretary, the operating room staff, the clinic staff, and the emergency room personnel. Remember, I considered returning there one day, so I didn't want to burn any bridges. But it wasn't meant to be.

That afternoon, on my final appearance in the orthopedic clinic, I received another phone call. "Dr. Mays, it's Dr. Smooth from Aggie University on the phone for you," the receptionist told me. Now what? "Well, Dr. Mays, have you thought about our offer?" I told him that if I didn't get into a four-year program, I was doing my residency in Arizona. "You can have your wish," he said. "I received notice today from a young man we had accepted into the residency program who's not going to join us. We discussed your proposal this morning at our faculty meeting and decided that rather than lose you, we would accept you this year. Frankly, we didn't feel you would come if we waited another year," Dr. Smooth explained.

My God, I had done it. I had won. My persistence had paid off. They took my bluff. Except it wasn't a bluff. I never would have returned to Aggie University. But now I would. To save a year of hell and sleepless nights on call, I would do almost anything. I told Dr. Smooth I was ecstatic and I accepted.

"I'll be home on Monday and I look forward to thanking you personally. I know you went to bat for me," I said. I knew, however, this wasn't true. Rather, time was drawing short and he needed a full quorum of residents in the program. He didn't want to look bad. After all, being a resident short would not look good with the high-powered national residency program committee which annually reviewed each program's certification.

Now came the hard part. How would I tell Dr. Flaps? I had developed an attachment to this man and I really didn't know how to say thanks, but no thanks. But I did. I found him in his office before lunch and told him the news. It was difficult. I explained to him I really wanted to train under him and I would have, had it not been for the incredible offer by Aggie University. He told me he was disappointed, but he understood and wished me luck. I felt empty and sad as I left his office. This was supposed to be one of the happiest days of my life. As I said good-bye to the residents and staff, it was clear I was leaving a place that really wanted me. And I wanted them.

I found my wife at the pool when I went home before lunch to tell her the news. She was excited that our future children would be raised near their grandparents. She ran to the phone to call her mother. I hustled to the swank restaurant for my departing lunch.

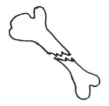

8. Residency

ON YOUR MARK, get set, go. The first day of my residency was, as you would imagine, both wonderful and frightening. I was "stoked" because I had made it. I had done the impossible. I was accepted into a four-year residency program right out of medical school instead of the more accepted five-year stint. I felt on top of the world. But let there be no mistake. I knew everyone out there would be watching me and looking for the "wonder boy" to make a mistake. They would be gunning for me. Would I let down the university? I was ready to be humble. I had worked hard for this achievement and I simply would not fail. I had won the initial game of medical school and I was prepared to make good on my next venture. I would just have to grin and bear the multiple jerks I encountered over the next few months who stabbed, "So you're the hot shot boy in orthopedics?"

We were first subjected to a meeting with Dr. Buttons, the chief of orthopedic surgery, who welcomed all the residents and told us how happy he was we were there. I believed he was sincere and obviously a gentleman. He assured us that if we had any problems to let him know. He said he would always be available to us.

We were then introduced to our chief residents. I was lucky to get this friendly guy from Texas, Dr. Boots. He had a great Southern accent and was very easygoing and thoroughly likable. Clearly he was a lucky draw for me. Why? Because the other chief resident was apparently in hot water with the entire faculty over several issues, including his marginal competence, and I was glad I wasn't in the middle of that Waterloo.

Dr. Boots was honest with me. He knew I had done some orthopedic work in Arizona, but he told me I was still the low man on the totem pole. I was in charge of all the scut work, like changing the casts on the ward patients, seeing to it that all the blood work was drawn before surgery, and making sure that the patients' consent forms were properly signed. "You see, Dr. Mays, we all had to do this when we first started, so you do too," he said. But that seemed fair enough to me.

Rounds on orthopedics were a great adventure. I referred to them as lightning rounds, because we didn't spend more than two minutes with each patient. "Good morning, Mrs. Dukas. How do you feel? Can you wiggle your toes? Fine. Get up with crutches today and if you're walking well by tomorrow, you can go home," Dr. Boots told a patient on the first day of rounds.

We were like a herd of cattle, like a wagon train. Next room. "Good morning, Mrs. Horland. I'm going to pull this small drain out of your hip now. It will burn just a little bit." (Like a towering inferno.) "Let's check your blood count today and get you up in a chair, okay?" Dr. Boots asked. Before she answered, we were out the door.

Everyone on rounds had a designated job. As the chief resident, Dr. Boots led the group. He was interested in only one thing: debriding the service (getting people out of the hospital), thus making rounds shorter. He was responsible for everyone on our team, including the junior residents (second- and third-year residents), the interns, the medical students, and, of course, the patients. He tried to alert us to the likes and dislikes of the professors so we would look good when they came with us on rounds about once a week. He lectured, "Dr. Buttons likes to know the patient's temperature, so make sure you're ready with the answer. And don't tell him the patient doesn't have a temperature. Every patient has a temperature. They may not have a fever, but just tell him the number. You know, like 98.6 or 100.2."

Later in clinic I had a chance to talk with Dr. Boots personally. He remembered me from medical school and promised I would be able do a lot of cases even as a first-year resident. "You're lucky," he said, "because I've already done a lot of surgery, I can hand down a significant amount of work to you and the junior resident." Such a deal. I was excited.

He encouraged me to get to know the faculty members, as they would make or break me over the next four years. He told me to read the orthopedic journal and to keep abreast of the current orthopedic literature. He emphasized how good residents looked when quoting a recent article. "And don't commit the ultimate sin: Don't ever make a professor look bad or make it appear that you know more than he does. Clam up in those instances."

Clinic was routine. Patients with fractures were everywhere. The idea was to get them in and out as fast as possible so we could go home. Initially I went over the cases with either Dr. Boots or the junior resident, Dr. Frito, but soon I could manage on my own and started directing traffic myself.

The clinics were also staffed by orthopedic surgeons from the community and it was politically expedient to present some of the cases to them too. This was for a couple of reasons. First, these doctors donated their time to the residents for educational reasons. Second, they were checking out the current crop of residents to see who might be good enough to be invited into the community upon completion of their residency.

We had some doozies. There was Dr. Law, whose character was only surpassed by his height. He was five feet tall. He tried to be impressive by always presenting an easier way for treating orthopedic injuries. "I have this trick that I use when I wrap on a hanging arm cast so that the sling never slips off the patient's arm," Dr. Law told us. He then showed us how he wound a piece of plaster around his fingers while casting a patient so that the patient could use the hole for a sling. We had to listen. We had no choice. "In surgery I find it difficult to hold two bones together in an open fracture. Since it's not legally wise to put foreign materials, such as plates, in contaminated wounds, I use a large suture that can't be seen on an x-ray (or in court) to tie the bones together. The attorneys never know," he chuckled.

I'd been warned about this guy. He was the local orthopedic legal prostitute. He testified in court at least once a week and had the reputation that if the pay was right, he would testify to whatever was necessary to keep in good graces with the local attorneys. He made a good living doing it and he paid little malpractice insurance because he wasn't operating. No one in town sent referrals to him because he was so busy testifying.

It took a special breed to do this kind of work, a man with

patience. When Dr. Law booked himself out of the office all day for a court appearance and the attorney called to say the case was settled, he didn't get angry. On another case he might meet for three to four hours the day before the court date. The morning of the trial, the attorney would call an hour before Dr. Law was scheduled to testify, informing him that there were no court rooms available. He learned to accept this. That's legal medicine.

I had been on the service for two weeks and I still hadn't done any surgery. But I wasn't worried. I was doing a lot of assisting in surgery and getting to know the ropes. The orthopedic technician in surgery was an elderly black lady who handed the residents the instruments they needed, not necessarily what they requested. "You ain't putting a three-eighths-inch drill in that bone. You drill a quarter inch like everybody else," she screeched.

Whenever I operated with a faculty member, I kept my mouth shut unless asked a question. I was there to learn. The professors usually operated only with a senior resident. If this resident wanted to hand the case to a more junior resident, the professor would merely come in and sign the chart without ever participating in, or even watching, the surgery.

The hospital couldn't be paid for the case unless a faculty member signed the chart, regardless of who operated on the patient. This was true even at three o'clock in the morning. The professor had to get out of bed and make an appearance at the hospital. The nurse carried the chart to the front desk so the professor could remain in street clothes to sign it and then leave, never seeing the patient or the procedure being done. He never met the patient. He never saw the x-rays.

Oh sure, the most senior resident had called to say, "Hi, Dr. Spud, sorry to bother you so late at night, but I have a thirty-five-year-old dirt ball who was shot in the leg by his girlfriend tonight when she caught him in bed with another woman. We thought we would go in and debride the wound and leave it open since there was no fracture," the resident explained. Usually the faculty member asked, "What time did you say it was? Never mind, go ahead and do what you think is right. I'll sign the chart in the morning."

But then the university would not get paid. Obviously, for the financial survival of the university, it was only a matter of time until the chairman of the orthopedics department insisted that all faculty members hustle in to sign the chart no matter what time of the day or night. He reminded all of the professors that it would be tough for them to get their yearly raises without their cooperation. I could never figure out how anyone would know when the chart was signed. Come in at 8:00 a.m. and write 3:00 a.m. Big deal, who would know?

Night call at the county hospital in orthopedics was a mess. All the solid citizens came out to play: the criminals who liked to donate their bodies to science, and the drunks who were so intoxicated they fell asleep with their arms and legs underneath them, only to awaken the next morning with a numb hand or dead foot. There were also the drug abusers who shot up with dirty needles, getting their arms so infected that they came into the emergency room with fevers up to 105 degrees and pus draining out of their skin.

As in Arizona, the more experience I acquired and the more my senior resident saw my work, the more he trusted me and gave me more responsibility. What this really translated into was that the senior resident could comfortably sneak home after the faculty left at night and cover me from home. Of course if I made a wrong decision or something didn't go according to plan, it was his ass and he knew it. But because of my significant orthopedic training before residency, I was given this luxury early in my first year.

The night I got my first surgical case was memorable. I was sitting in the residents' office about 9:30 p.m. and began dozing while studying the orthopedic journal. My beeper went off and it was the emergency room doctor saying he had a thirty-seven-year-old female who had tried to commit suicide by jumping out the third floor of her house. She failed—to kill herself, that is. She did manage to fracture her hip. This was a relatively uncommon injury in a young person.

I wandered down to see this unfortunate lady. It was as advertised: a scared young female who had a painful, malaligned lower extremity. X-rays confirmed her fractured hip. I called my senior resident at home to tell him about the patient. He told me to admit her to the hospital and, since he was tired of fixing hips, this was my case. Holy Toledo! I was only a brand-new, first-year resident and I was going to get to pin a hip. This was an orthopedist's dream. It's the bread-and-butter operation we do.

I hurried back to the patient to calmly tell her that she had broken her hip and that she would need surgery. As I explained the procedure and its risks to her, I couldn't help but lick my lips with excitement at my very first surgical case. But I realized after several moments that this poor lady had no idea what I was saying. She was frightened and confused. She had just tried to kill herself. She didn't care about her hip. I decided to talk to her later. I admitted her to the ward with plenty of medication for sleep, pain, and agitation.

Remembering all I had learned about caring for the total patient, I phoned the psychiatric resident on call and asked if one of the psychiatrists from the rather low-keyed psychiatric crisis clinic could stop by and see if this patient needed special attention, drugs, or restraining. We couldn't admit her to the psychiatric ward as she had an acute surgical problem, and it might freak out all the crazies on the psychiatric ward. Can you imagine what these people would think if they saw a patient hung up in traction ropes and slings? The psychiatrist called me later to say she needed heavy sedation and restraints because she could try suicide again, although even he admitted it would be hard for her to walk to the window and jump with a broken hip.

After I dictated a short note on her admission, I ran back to the residents' office and studied the text on hip fractures and how to fix them. I had helped on several types of hip fractures already, but now I was going to get to do the cutting. In addition, I knew that I would be questioned tomorrow about the type of fracture and the best fixation and all the recent articles in the literature. So I said the hell with sleeping for now and readied myself for tomorrow's rounds.

Later, as I lay in bed, I planned my incision. I didn't want to go too fast, as I knew I should control all the bleeding. Then I would put a guide pin up the neck and head of the femur bone, use a big drill measured at just the right length for the right size screw, and fasten the side plate to the bone with a clamp. It would be a cinch. Or would it? What could go wrong? Would I have trouble getting the guide pin in straight? No, that would be easy. I realized I didn't quite understand how to measure for the right screw distance into the head, so I quickly turned on the light and studied that portion of the procedure. The rest should be easy. I'd use good technique and go slowly, I wouldn't be clumsy, and I'd be patient with the nurses.

The next morning on rounds, the chief resident and the junior resident were more benign than I had anticipated. They had seen the x-rays before rounds and knew it was a simple intertrochanteric fracture of the hip. "You've seen us fix these, so this should be easy for you," Dr. Frito, the junior resident kidded. All that studying was worth it because I learned a few things I had taken for granted. Besides, it was early and the faculty could still challenge me. The surgery was added to the schedule for 5:00 p.m., after clinic.

The day went by without incident. That was fine with me since I wasn't interested in too much publicity for my first operation, in case something went wrong. I arrived in surgery a half hour early to make sure all the equipment was ready and the fracture table was set up properly. I was taught that the surgeon was the captain of the ship. If something went wrong or something wasn't ready, it would be my fault.

I was excited when the patient arrived, though she didn't appear very enthused. We got her into the operating room and put her to sleep. We didn't feel this lady was a good candidate for a spinal anesthetic because the noise of the tools and the drills might make this rather unstable personality even more so. She was moved onto the fracture table and I reduced her hip. X-rays were taken to see if the fracture was well aligned. Damn! The reduction wasn't adequate. I needed to improve it significantly before my chief resident showed up. I adjusted the foot, applied more traction, and re-x-rayed the hip, but it still looked bad.

Then Dr. Boots came through the door. "Things are all set up, but I'm not happy with my reduction," I said. He showed me that I had fastened the foot strap incorrectly onto the fracture table and that I needed more traction. I could see this was routine for him and what he said made sense.

After his adjustments, the x-rays looked good, so we went out to scrub our hands. I started to feel like a real surgeon. I was lucky to have an understanding senior resident. He reviewed the technique while we scrubbed. The case went smoothly. It took thirty-five minutes and the fixation looked good. As soon as I started sewing the skin Dr. Boots told me I had done a nice job and he left. That showed confidence. After the dressing was on, I thanked everyone for being patient with me, and I left the room feeling like a real surgeon. I had operated. I had called the shots. It was me who had asked for the instruments. Lift off.

Initially, I hadn't cared that this lady was emotionally disturbed. She had a legitimate orthopedic problem and I was able to fix it. But I was also her doctor. I came back to the hospital after dinner that evening even though I was not on call. I wanted to see my patient. I had operated on her. Her ability to walk was in my hands. She was doing fine. She had a slight fever, which was normal after surgery, but other than that she was wiggling her toes on the operated leg.

The next morning I went to see her before rounds and her hip looked fine. Actually, as it turned out, this lady was just going through a severely emotional time and she was very nice. She appeared more stable than her history indicated. We talked easily. After a few days, she was up on crutches and making good progress with physical therapy. Dr. Frito reminded me, "When a patient with a hip fracture can get up and walk on her own, out the door she goes. Ready or not. There are too many patients on the ward, so let's clear out the service." I told him that I would get her out as quickly as possible.

But wait a minute. Was this lady emotionally stable? Was I about to win the battle and lose the war? She wouldn't leave the hospital and do something foolish again, or would she? I decided to go back to the room, pull up a chair, sit down, and have a heart-to-heart chat with her. She didn't really talk openly about her personal situation or her suicide attempt, but it seemed as though her support group at home would be strong enough to keep tabs on her. I decided I would speak to her family before discharging her.

On my way over to the clinic, I noticed the chief of the psychiatric consult service walking across the lawn. I flagged her down and explained my predicament. She agreed it might be wise to stop by, with her residents and students, of course, and see if I should release this potential keg of dynamite to the real world. This was known in the business as covering your ass. If they saw her, said she was okay, and wrote a note to that effect in her chart, I'd be covered legally if she tried suicide again. But I cared more deeply for the patient than that. This was my first hip fracture. I wanted to see it heal and have the patient do well. I wanted her to walk normally again.

The next morning I arrived at the hospital early and went to the ward to review the psychiatric consult note. They felt comfortable discharging the patient and agreed her family support group was adequate to help prevent further suicide attempts. They made an appointment for her to return to the psychiatric clinic in one week for follow-up.

The orthopedic team bid her farewell on rounds and I stayed behind to tell her that if she had any problems at all, to please call me. I even gave her my home telephone number. (I would be cured of this bad habit quickly.) I reassured her that she had done very well, considering the situation, and that she was lucky to have a second chance. I was delighted that my first surgery had gone without a hitch and the victim left the hospital alive. I hoped the rest of my career would be so successful.

I turned my attention toward the other patients on the ward now that my patient was gone. The entire day was spent in surgery and I helped on a large spine case which took four hours. This was followed by a typical county hospital patient who had multiple injuries from a motorcycle accident. We were called in to splint the multiple fractures in his arms and legs while the neurosurgeons opened up his head to drain out the huge blood clots that would ultimately make him a gork, if he lived.

The next morning I prepared for x-ray conference and got to the conference room early to make sure the x-rays were ready. I couldn't wait to show them off. They were beautiful. The pin was in perfect position. They'd better be impressed. I felt so good that I ran across the street to grab a doughnut at the local hospital hangout. As I stood in line waiting to pay I glanced at the front page of the newspaper held by a nurse in front of me. My stomach began to churn. It couldn't possibly be. The headline on the front page read: "Woman Jumps to Her Death off Hotel Roof." Please let it be somebody else. This is just a coincidence. The nurse let me look closer. I was devastated, it was my patient. I had let her go. I had killed her.

I couldn't decide what to do at x-ray conference. Should I tell the faculty and residents at conference about her death? I knew the right thing to do was to discuss the situation with Dr. Boots. He urged me to forget it and tell the faculty later. He agreed that we had done the right thing and many people would not have even gotten the psychiatric consultation in the first place. All the residents and faculty applauded my efforts at conference and assured me my hip pinning was beautifully accomplished. But I felt completely destroyed.

After the conference, I called the chief of the psychiatric consult services and told her the grim news. She was in disbelief. She had seen the patient herself, hadn't even pawned the case off to one of her residents or students. She apologized and said, "These things happen." I'm sure they do.

That afternoon in clinic I was useless. I wondered if all of my surgical cases were going to end in catastrophe. I felt like I had done a great job but had failed. I was called by the chief of pathology services who did the autopsies for the hospital. The patient was taken to our county hospital for an autopsy because of the suicide. The chart was reviewed and the pathologist wanted my input on the case. I told him the whole story and he agreed it was unfortunate, but what else could I have done as her surgeon? As I was about to hang up the phone, I told him I had a ridiculous request. "I wonder if you could do an x-ray in the morgue of her left hip and see how my hip pinning fared in the fall?" I asked.

"Probably not very good after an eight-story fall. But I'm looking at it on the slab as we speak and it looks straight. I'll take an x-ray," he said.

You won't believe it. The fixation held perfectly and none of the screws or the plate was broken. Somehow this news didn't make me feel any better.

The remainder of my first year was merely a matter of survival. Residency was not supposed to be fun, I know. It was just getting patients in and out of the hospital and hopefully learning something along the way. My first year was devoted to being an errand boy for the staff and senior residents. But I wanted to graduate to the second year, so I never made waves or refused to accommodate. If I did my life would have been made miserable, whether I deserved it or not.

But how did you learn? There were several ways you tried. You could read the orthopedic journal. There were two problems with this. I was normally so tired by the time I escaped home that the last thing I wanted to do was read, especially the journal. Most of us were married, and had to pay bills, water the lawn, and be with our families. The other problem with the journal was that it contained mostly irrelevant articles that had nothing to do with the everyday office orthopedic practice.

It was filled with articles about things most orthopedists had never seen and never would, like "The incidence of curved spines in Orientals living under tents" or "The peculiar blood supply of the tibia seen in the left legs of Doberman pinschers." Once in a blue moon something pertinent was published.

You have to remember who was writing this junk. Remember those professors in college and medical school, publish or perish? This was the same scene. They had to write a bunch of meaningless articles or find another job. So they all wrote and wrote. The material didn't have to be interesting or relevant. Of course those who sat on committees were all in a conspiracy with each other so they could keep their comfortable jobs at the universities. It was a big joke.

There were a few other journals that were published by practicing physicians. The articles were generally more useful and stimulating. I have published in these magazines with great success and interest from the readers.

During my residency, there were monthly journal clubs we were forced to attend. Normally these were held at the home of a bone setter in private practice. This was good because at least they would provide some good eats. For two hours one of our own university professors lectured on the more salient points of journal articles. The only saving grace was that after the lecture was over and the faculty member left, the host would reassure the residents that all the professors were full of shit, and we would never have to worry about any of this nonsense.

It became obvious to me that the best way to learn the trade was from the more senior residents. They learned the tricks with time and hopefully passed them down. I was lucky that mine did. He steered me toward the classic articles in the literature and I began to keep files on them.

Oh, and don't think for one minute we were done with taking tests. Every year there was the famed in-service exam that would test our knowledge against the other residents across this great land. This was where I made one of the greatest mistakes of my training.

It was a tactical error. I had been told repeatedly that the faculty put a lot of emphasis on the in-service results and I should go out of my way to look good. I was advised to study a few weeks before the exam and look at some of the old tests to see the sort of questions they asked. I was told that if you scored badly, make sure you did it the first year and improved every year after that. That way the faculty would think you were learning each year and that they were teaching you well.

I had so much orthopedic exposure before my residency that I scored in the upper five percent of the first-year residents across the country. Big mistake. My second-year scores were lower than my first year and my third-year scores were lower than my second. And yes, my senior-year scores dropped so low that I was warned by the department head that there was a good chance I wouldn't pass the orthopedic board exam at the end of my residency. Screw 'em if they can't take a joke.

My second year was a little less stressful than my first. I was able to concentrate more on studying and surgery because my first-year resident took over the dirty work.

The weekly x-ray conferences were very stimulating. Each week the residents got together with the faculty and discussed all the orthopedic patients currently in the hospital. The chairman of the department would sit in the front row because he was supposed to be the smartest and the one with the most experience. Dr. Buttons was exactly that, so it wasn't a problem. The hand surgeon, Dr. Pipe, sat toward the back because he smoked. Most of the hand stuff was done on an outpatient basis anyway, so there wasn't much for him to show off. After all, this really was show-and-tell.

The chief of the spine service, Dr. Spud, showed the preoperative x-rays of a young girl with a severe 85-degree scoliosis curve before surgery. It was corrected to 15 degrees on her postoperative film. I must admit these x-rays were impressive, with large hooks and rods holding the spine straight. Nobody minded verbally patting Dr. Spud on the back because he was a nice guy and did very good work. He liked to play sports with the other residents and came across as a friend.

Then there was Dr. Rail, our staff man who professed to be an expert on children's orthopedics. He thought he was cool because he had long hair and an impressive mustache, but he was considered a jerk by all, including the nurses. The thing about Dr. Rail that always amused me was that he professed to be good at all aspects of orthopedics. Clearly he was not good at any aspect. He came from a prestigious residency that was famous for orthopedic pathology and academics but where they virtually saw no trauma whatsoever. When a trauma case was discussed, he was the first to criticize the care and brag about the number of legs he had fixed so much better than we. It was sickening. He was obviously lying. Many of his cases went to hell with his management.

Dr. Smooth was a social climber and the head of the total joint service. He put in new joints faster than lightning. He trained you if he liked you, or if there was something you might potentially offer him in the future, or if you patronized him.

His friend, Dr. Nadaworda, spoke English so poorly he could hardly be understood. We took his lectures as gospel and said thank you very much. But he was a good surgeon and if you went to the operating room with him, he could teach you some good techniques.

During the second year we rotated through the Free For All Clinic. This was a local prepaid health plan with plenty of patients and good bread-and-butter orthopedics. There were about ten orthopedists on staff, and they were as different as day and night.

The chief orthopedist was a true character. Dr. Mac was a very nice man, but he talked too much. If you wanted to do a straightforward operation like putting a total hip in a patient with severe arthritis, he would ask whether all forms of conservative treatment had been tried. If you wanted to change a cast on a baby's foot each week, he would ask you how fast a baby's foot grows. None of these questions were unreasonable, but they were asked just to let us know that he was the professor and we were the grunts.

The other members of Dr. Mac's staff were all partners in this health system, so they loved residents. Why? Because they made the same amount of money no matter how much they worked or how many surgeries they completed. So if they could get the residents to see the patients, do all the preoperative workups, make rounds on their patients, and dictate all the reports, they could sit in their big offices and smoke cigarettes all day. They gladly gave up the good surgical cases just to get out of the work associated with them. And they left promptly at 4 p.m. each day.

Staff members were constantly approaching me in the hallway and begging, "I have a guy in my office with a locked knee that needs surgery. If you want to work him up, you can do the surgery." For a hungry second-year resident, this was heaven. I ended up working long hours, but I did a lot of surgery and gained incredible experience. I gladly played the game on this rotation and was hassled infrequently unless I operated with Dr. Mac. He meant well, but just carried it to an extreme. And was he slow. If I had a case with him it was best to have a nurse start an IV in my arm prior to the surgery so I could be fed intravenously during the event. There would certainly be no lunch and maybe no dinner.

The staff at the Free For All Clinic had no interest in taking call. They had made enough money over the years that they gladly paid the residents rotating through the service to take their call in the emergency room. I did it gladly. I could make more in an evening than I made all month as a resident at the county hospital. If I wanted to take an entire weekend, I could be rich! Since much of the call could be handled from home, I would have been stupid not to oblige.

During my third year of residency it was evident to me I would receive adequate training but certainly not an outstanding amount. Why? Because our program needed much more input from the private practicing physicians in the community. They were the guys who did the everyday stuff like the knee ligament and total joint surgeries, and the shoulder reconstructions. The professors at the university didn't know anything about these procedures. What was worse, the professors were very poor operating surgeons. They were poor technicians. But the third year allowed us to spend three months at the community hospitals with the private doctors.

But things began looking up. The chairman of the department called an emergency meeting to tell us some news, wonderful for everybody, I thought. Dr. Smooth had just accepted an offer to become chairman of the department of orthopedics at a Southern university. He was going to take Dr. Pipe and Dr. Nadaworda with him, leaving the program only three faculty members. This meant there were too few professors to supervise the residents. He said he would entertain any reasonable proposal for us to spend time away from the program as long as the elective was in a quality institution with quality people, by university standards, of course.

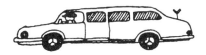

9. Dr. Rosey

THE WHEELS of fortune started turning in my brain. I had this dream about spending some time with a sports doctor, so I decided to make some phone calls, even if my chances were slim to none. I felt that this would be the fad of the future, because sports medicine was growing in popularity. The local professional football team seemed like a good place to start. Shoot for the moon, right? I phoned the team's main office to obtain the name of their orthopedic surgeon. I was confused as they explained that Dr. Rosey lived in Southern California, four hundred miles away from the team. How could this be?

I made a long-distance phone call to Dr. Rosey. I was given his office manager, Hilda. She presented like a fullback. "I'm wondering if there's any chance I could come to your office and spend a few months with Dr. Rosey?" I asked. I explained that I had heard many great things about Dr. Rosey and I just wanted to learn from the best. People complain that they are in the wrong place at the wrong time. I wasn't.

She told me that Dr. Rosey had never had a resident or a student in his office and he was not affiliated with any university. Furthermore, he was a very busy man and really didn't have time to teach. But I was sensing some thought going on in her head as she spoke. Apparently, one of Dr. Rosey's partners was about to leave the office and an extra hand might be helpful. She agreed that the idea was far-fetched, but she would talk to Dr. Rosey and get back to me soon. I reassured her that I would give anything for this experience and that

I would work day and night if required. Somehow I felt optimistic by her tone and decided not to pursue any other avenues until I heard from her.

Between surgery cases that afternoon, I noted a message on the door for me. Hilda had called from Dr. Rosey's office and wanted to speak to me immediately. I was so excited I could hardly talk. I anticipated a yes vote. I told the first-year resident to get started with the next case if I didn't get back in time, even though it was a case I very much wanted to do. I ran up the stairs of the hospital, three floors to the residents' office, to call Hilda. She said she had spoken with Dr. Rosey and he agreed to my idea. She asked me when I would be able to come and I told her I just did.

I said I would have to talk to the chairman of my department, but I thought I'd be available within a few weeks. Hilda encouraged me to arrive as soon as possible, now that Dr. Rosey was shorthanded. She alluded to the fact that his partner was leaving under unpleasant circumstances, but I didn't want to get into that. And then came the good stuff. She had thought about where I could live. It seemed that Dr. Rosey's sister was a real estate broker, and she listed a condo on the beach at Marina. Dr. Rosey's office would pay for this in exchange for my working in his office. In addition, Hilda had talked to a friend of hers who worked at Oscar Hospital, which had a fund to pay visiting house staff. Had I died and gone to heaven? Was this conversation really taking place?

And last but not least, she talked about the football team. Dr. Rosey realized the reason I called him was to, in some way, be involved in sports medicine. He promised to get me involved as much as possible with the team, but he couldn't guarantee that I would travel to the games or even be on the sidelines. I wanted to say all the right things, so I reiterated I would do whatever was asked of me. If I couldn't be with Dr. Rosey at the games, I would gladly stay behind and take his call at the hospital. But there was hope because he had one other associate in the office who didn't care much for sports. Maybe he would take the bulk of the responsibility during the football season.

I ran down the ramp so excitedly that I sprained my ankle. I limped back into the operating room where the resident was wrist-deep in a hip incision. But I let him finish the case and kept my excitement to myself until I had a chance to talk to Dr. Buttons. After the case, I rushed over to see him in his office and was told he was in clinic. I strolled down there to find him writing in a chart.

He started telling me about a young girl with a unique orthopedic elbow problem that had been referred to him from one hundred miles away. He wondered if I would like to go in to see the patient with him. I was delighted, of course. After spending fifteen minutes with this uninteresting problem, Dr. Buttons and I left the room. He finally asked me what I was doing in clinic with my scrub suit on. I said that I wanted to talk with him and I offered to wait until he was finished seeing patients.

Since that had been his last patient, he invited me to go back into the lounge and sit down. After he shut the door, I explained my incredible find to him. He didn't say no, but he wanted to talk to Dr. Rosey because he was concerned that there was no university affiliation. He didn't just want to lose track of a resident for six months. But I knew Dr. Buttons well. He sensed one of his residents might be exposed to the big time and this, in turn, might in some way reflect brightly on his program. Possibly one of his residents might be seen on the sidelines on national television. Whoopee! He agreed to chat with Dr. Rosey by phone the next day. I furnished him with the number and it was just then I realized that I still had not spoken to Dr. Rosey either.

I anticipated I would get the go-ahead, so I began to sort through the problems of leaving for six months, like my six-week surgery schedule and my house being vacant. Could I rent it? But then I realized that none of these items were as important as the opportunity that lay in front of me. I was ready. The next day in clinic, I received a call from Hilda, who boasted how she and Dr. Rosey had buttered up Dr. Buttons. They had assured him that the experience I would receive would be outstanding and that Oscar Hospital was indeed affiliated with the local university medical center. Once again, as after my residency acceptance, I was basking in glory. I felt I had conquered another hurdle on just a whim, by making just one phone call.

Before my conversation ended with Hilda, I asked her if I might speak with Dr. Rosey before I showed up at his front door. She agreed that this seemed only fair, even though he was a busy celebrity, and the orthopedist for a dynamic and successful professional football team.

He called me at home that evening and was not what I had imagined. He sounded very elderly and distant, almost confused. He mentioned that he had just seen his last patient in the office. I looked at the clock and noticed it was 8:45 p.m. Was this common to be seeing patients at this time of night? Would I be doing this every night? He sounded like a genuinely nice man and he was looking forward to having me in his office. He said he knew I would probably like to come to some of the games and he promised he would talk to the owner about this. At the very least, he would be able to get me a seat in the stands and I could join him in the locker room before and after the games. I ended the conversation by telling him I knew he was very busy and that I appreciated his taking a few minutes to return my call. I reconfirmed my dedication to hard work. I couldn't wait to get there.

He admitted he had always wanted to do some teaching and that everyone else in Southern California always seemed to get all of the sports medicine press because they were in a university setting. I quipped that maybe we could make some headlines of our own. He seemed to like that. I mentioned I had some experience in writing articles and maybe we could publish a few papers together. He became even more excited. He ended up by asking me if I thought this one-bedroom condominium on the beach would suffice for my family. I told him I thought I could tolerate it for a few months.

It was arranged that we would meet with Dr. Rosey's sister, the realtor, when we arrived in Southern California. I quickly finished my obligations at the university. We let one of the medical students use our house and off we went. As we entered the intimidating Southern California metropolis, we followed the signs to Marina. It was a rather tacky little hippie-type village but the beauty of the ocean took precedence. We were running late, so we asked directions to our temporary residence and our excitement mounted as we were told it was on the street that ran along the beach.

When we finally arrived, I ran up to the mailbox area and called to the room. This was exclusive. You couldn't just bolt upstairs. Dr. Rosey's sister answered my buzz and came down to welcome us. She showed me how to use the appropriate keys and the garage door opener, bid us farewell and good luck. Then we finally had a chance to relax. The living room window allowed an incredible view of the Pacific Ocean. The back door opened directly onto the warm sand. I liked this job already.

Even though it was Sunday, after I finished unpacking I called Dr. Rosey. His exchange said he would be roaming around on call and to beep him when we arrived. Thirty minutes later he answered my beep and we agreed to meet at the hospital in an hour. He would meet my family later.

As I was leaving, I paused in the garage to chat with another tenant. His tall frame and face looked familiar. Then I realized he played professional basketball for the Southern California Smog. I asked for the quickest way to Rodeo Hills, for both that day and during the week, because I was sure there was going to be unforgettable traffic. I told him how impressed I was to be living in the same building with such a celebrity. He invited me to go jogging in the mornings with him and several real movie stars he was sure I would instantly recognize. They lived on the same street. I was having fun now.

I found my way to the hospital and asked for directions to the orthopedic ward. I looked around and asked where I might find Dr. Rosey. The nurse said he was just there and had probably gone into a patient's room. Then he appeared, a man that would change the course of my life. He greeted me with a warm smile. He was more elderly than I had imagined. He was very small, a little hard-of-hearing, and seemed quite laid-back. He invited me to walk across the street for lunch.

I knew instantly this was going to be wonderful. Dr. Rosey seemed somewhat lonely but with a heart of gold. He said he lived at home some of the time. Although he and his wife were technically married, they weren't really. We both talked about our expectations. He told me of the recent unpleasant departure of his partner and how I had come along at the right time. He mentioned I would get to do a lot of assisting in surgery and after I was comfortable I could see patients in the office. In addition, the football team was currently practicing in Southern California for the upcoming preseason and having daily scrimmages. He said if I weren't busy I could run out there with him later that afternoon. You bet.

As we drove out to the scrimmage, he asked if I had any sports medicine experience. I embarrassedly told him that I had stood on many sidelines at high school football games. He assured me that professional football was somewhat different. He warned me that I would not be well accepted at first by the players or management. He said, "Keep your distance and mind your own business. After a while, they'll be more comfortable with you."

When we arrived at camp, I could immediately see his point. The players all greeted him and looked at me very critically. But I was in "hog heaven." I was here with athletes I had read about and cheered for over the years. Dr. Rosey was very good about introducing me to everybody. I felt like a kid in a candy store.

The coach was everything I thought he would be and more. He was a big teddy bear. He didn't pay much attention to me, but I just stared at him. He was fascinating. He was so huge. But his face looked like he had coached for fifty years.

And then, as I was listening to the latest injury report, I saw him out of the corner of my eye. He was heading our way. My palms started to sweat. It was the owner. He looked like he was going to kill someone. And he looked right at me. I moved my position closer to my mentor. Dr. Rosey introduced me and the owner shook my hand as he looked somewhere else. He wasn't interested in me in the least. Thank God.

I went with Dr. Rosey to the training area, where he examined some players and good-naturedly joked with them. It was fun. One kidded him that the knee that he had operated on three times was still no good. "Is this elbow always going to be crooked?" the tight-end quipped. Another asked if it was time for another injection in his rib cage. I was fascinated. My first day was so stimulating I wondered how I would sleep that night.

On the drive back he talked about his fifteen years with the team, the good and the bad. He asked about my family. Even in the short time we had been together, I could feel a father-and-son relationship developing. He was at ease with me, partly because we were both Jewish. We talked of the politics in private practice and how everyone in town was jealous of him because he took care of the team. He warned me that I might hear negative things about him because of his status in the community, but I promised to be thick-skinned and "true to my school."

I rushed back to the beach to find my wife and child out on the sand enjoying their new paradise. I raved about my first day and suggested we go out to dinner to celebrate. This would be the greatest elective known to residents. All from a simple phone call. We took a walk on the beach while I boasted how I had met all the players I had been idolizing since my teen years.

The scene was unbelievable. The ocean was fifty yards from our back door and the beach was filled with volleyball nets. We even had our own pier. We were within walking distance of all the little shops in the village. The beautiful blond star of a popular comedy series lived right next door to us. We went to a restaurant that evening to finalize a most memorable day. It had started at 6:00 a.m. with an eight-hour drive. I started feeling good again.

I got up early the next morning to make sure I didn't get caught in traffic. I took the street route into Rodeo Hills, which turned out to be excellent advice. I entered the parking garage at the office and was happy to find the attendant had heard I was coming to join Dr. Rosey. I had my own parking space next to Dr. Rosey. How much better could this get?

Even though I was an hour early, Hilda was there. She was as advertised. A large woman, very young, and she frightened me. I thought she was going to hurt me. She invited me to sit down in her office. She was nice, but firm, as she explained how the office worked, our schedule, and what she visualized my role to be. She bluntly said to me that if I did a good job and Dr. Rosey liked me, I would probably be able to travel with him to all of the games. She implied she had influence with the team administration and might be inclined to use it if I performed up to her expectations. I got her message: She ran the office, plain and simple. I didn't answer to Dr. Rosey, I answered to her. If I had a problem, I was to come to her. If it happened that I was a real star and might some day want to come to work in this office, she would make that decision. I was overwhelmed. But when I thought back to our conversation two weeks ago, it all came together. She had sized me up, figured I might have some usefulness to them in the office, and arranged for my visit.

She lectured that Dr. Rosey was very busy and that he got behind with his medical records and dictating at the hospital. I could help with that. She had checked with the hospital and I was approved to dictate his history and physicals, operative reports, and discharge summaries. She said I could help in the office by putting on casts, writing prescriptions, and making notes in the office charts. After my briefing I took a deep breath, wondering if I could survive this overwhelming woman. She quickly introduced me to the office staff, leading me around like a drill sergeant.

Dr. Rosey's remaining partner arrived and I could immediately see why he was there. He was very meek. Hilda interrupted us to tell him he was supposed to be in surgery. She pointed him out the door. Good-bye.

I went to check the daily office schedule and noticed appointments starting at 9:00 a.m. But my watch said 9:35 a.m. Where was Dr. Rosey? I remembered him calling me late at night two weeks ago when he had finally finished with patients. He showed up at 9:50 a.m., grabbed his white coat and said, "Let's get started."

I followed him around for the entire week. What an experience. He had incredible patients, the likes of which I had never seen. Some had been through four back operations. Old Jewish people, wearing more gold than I had ever seen, stopped in the office for a social visit. Some were movie stars I had watched on television for years. It was fascinating.

Dr. Rosey was very polite and talkative, which was why he was so far behind. He talked to them about their families and about last week's football game. His favorite thing was the patients telling him they had seen his face on television standing on the sidelines. He loved this. His eyes lit up. The football team was obviously his life, his reason to live.

His habitual lateness was difficult for me. I was taught to be on time. Dr. Rosey was never on time. He would tell me to meet him at 8:00 a.m. and he would show up at 8:45 a.m. to make rounds in the hospital. I would finish rounds on my own and then when he showed up, he would simply stop by and say hello to the patients. He didn't have to write any orders or notes as I had already completed this chore.

We arrived in surgery at least half an hour late. This, of course, made the operating room supervisor angry. But he got away with it because the supervisor was an avid football fan and he gave her free tickets to the games. He was charming. He called everybody honey.

The rooms in Dr. Rosey's office were small. They were equipped with the usual injectables, models of knees and backs, and suture removal instruments. You can imagine how crowded the room was with Dr. Rosey, me, the patient, and usually at least one other family member. The worst part was that each room had a wall telephone. This turned out to be a major source of tardiness. Every phone call Hilda deemed important was buzzed into the room. Right in the middle of a patient's history the phone would ring and Dr. Rosey would excuse himself to talk, right in front of everyone. It might have been someone from the football team or the training staff. But it was usually his broker or his bookie calling for Dr. Rosey's weekly picks. Occasionally it was the hospital. Then again, it could have been his wife. I could always tell when it was his wife because he would whisper and say, "Not right now, honey." I always tried to talk to the patients during his wife's calls because I was embarrassed for him. They were not close and she was a nag.

I made the mistake of telling Hilda that I thought most of these interruptions were unnecessary and that they put us even further behind. I said this only after she had told me that she wished Dr. Rosey could run on time. However, I think my remark definitely gave me a black mark with her. After all, these interruptions were one of her ways of staying in control. Only she had access to the doctor. She called the shots. There was no doubt.

I learned several good surgical tricks from Dr. Rosey. He had an incredible amount of experience with reconstructions of the knee and shoulder. He often let me do parts of these procedures and I became proficient at surgical techniques that would ultimately be very important to me in my career. His handling of tissues was rough and he was slow. But his ideas were good and his approach to athletic injuries was surgically aggressive.

Our results were variable. This was mainly because Dr. Rosey liked to do a lot of back surgery. Most of the knees and shoulders did well, but the backs were unpredictable, as with most back surgeries. I often questioned Dr. Rosey's indications for some of these repeat surgeries and this, too, put a black mark against me. As a person in training, I felt the need to ask such questions like, "Do you agree with the orthopedic literature which documents that every time a patient has another back operation, the chance of obtaining a good result lessens?"

In retrospect, I should've kept my mouth shut, as my questions couldn't do anything but cause antagonism. But I was the one who had to dictate the history and physical, and it was considered the standard of care to state the problem the patient had, what previous treatments he had had, and what you hoped to accomplish by the procedure. In other words, would it make sense to a committee reading this report that the procedure was necessary? If we had a complication or if the chart were brought up for review by the hospital quality assurance committee, these facts would be important. Remember what I said about covering your ass.

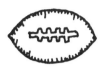

10. The Team

IT WORKED out that I could not only travel to the football games but be on the sidelines with Dr. Rosey. This first exposure to professional sports was the most incredible high of my life. Me actually mingling with these famous players and watching the world's most exciting sport from the best seat in the house! Dr. Rosey's rapport with the players was very good. I kept my distance, took in everything, and said nothing.

We had the same agenda each weekend, travelling to the away games by flying to Bayview to catch the team plane. Frequently Dr. Rosey was late and on two occasions the team plane had to wait for us. I felt bad because everyone looked at us critically and I worried they might think I had caused the delay.

We normally arrived two or three days before the away games. Dr. Rosey and I each had a private room. I was flying on a professional football team's chartered plane in first class and I stayed in my own room. Wow!

On the road I attended practice every day. Dr. Rosey usually went but not always. He often knew people in the cities where we played and was occasionally off on his own. But this wasn't all bad. If he were gone, the training staff would check an injury status with me and we ended up getting to know each other better.

The rest of the time before the game I was alone. I wandered around each city or watched television. At night Dr. Rosey had dinner with the owner and I wasn't invited.

On game day the pregame meal was four hours before kickoff. This was an incredible experience. Everyone wore his game face.

Don't smile, be uptight because we had a game to play and some asses to kick. Dr. Rosey and I sat at the table with the executive assistant and the head coach. Coach Hey often stared in my direction. This scared me because he was big, overpowering, and unpredictable.

One time when we were in Seattle, a former team doctor walked into the pregame meal room unannounced. He seemed to know almost everyone, and the guard at the door greeted him with a handshake and let him in. Coach Hey was furious. He jumped out of his chair and yelled to the guard to get this intruder out immediately. The coach explained afterward that this guy had been relieved of his duties several years ago because of strange religious behavior. I wondered if he liked me. I just didn't want him to hurt me.

The buses for the game left the hotel at 10:00 a.m. for the 1:00 p.m. game. I frequently rode the early bus because the players went then and I liked to watch them getting taped in the locker room. That was why I was there, to learn.

I gazed out the window, wondering when I would see the stadium. I loved looking at stadiums. They were massive, perfect, and round. I had watched them on T.V. for so many years that I wondered if they would really look as formidable. They didn't. They were much bigger.

When we arrived at the visitors' locker room, I stationed myself near the training tables to watch and experience this incredible art. Certain players insisted that only the head trainer tape their ankles. Some liked the younger assistant trainers. They all looked good to me.

When Dr. Rosey arrived it was time to evaluate certain players to see whether or not they were ready to play. This was often decided right before the game. "My knee felt fine in practice yesterday, Doc, but today it feels stiff." Usually the final decision was a combination of input from the trainer, the doctor, the player, and the coaches.

The coaches were all different. Some would say, "If you can't play one hundred percent, you don't play." Others would say, "Number eighty beat you so badly three weeks ago, you're probably afraid to go out and try to cover him today, you pussy." They were serious. I feared a fight would break out.

There were many rituals by the players. "Where's the gum?" one player yelled. Another insisted, "It's time for my vitamin B-12 shot." Some would go sit in the bathroom for an hour and read the game program. The quarterback, running back, wide receiver, and center played poker for an hour before the game. One player was accustomed to vomiting in the nearest garbage can after suiting up. He was a bundle of nerves and always looked anxious. One player with chronic rib pain would approach Dr. Rosey for his weekly injection. They would meet in a back room with a needle and syringe, out of everyone's view.

For pregame warm-up, the players would go out on the field without their shoulder pads in order to stretch, loosen up, run and pass the ball. The kickers would practice field goals and the receivers would run patterns.

I went just to look at the ballpark. My God, how massive! They usually held between 60,000 and 80,000 people. And here I was down on the field. I knew I was lucky and frequently told myself so. The owner came out to study his troops. He intently watched the drills of the other team, too. I retreated to the opposite end of the field so I would not be in his way, so he would not ask me anything. I was clearly afraid of him. And he knew it.

After thirty minutes the players returned to the locker room. It was time to get serious, to put on shoulder pads and tight jerseys, and to get air properly adjusted in their helmets. The players hit themselves hard on their helmets to make sure the amount of air was adequate. Coaches for each of the specialty teams reviewed the game plan with their squads. A player who needed immediate taping rushed into the training room, and some players consulted Dr. Rosey about last-minute drainage of fluid from their knees or other possible injections.

Then the referee entered the locker room and yelled, "Two minutes." The room became quiet. "Okay, listen up," Coach Hey barked. "Now all the preparation for this week is over and you all know your jobs. Defense has to tackle. Offense has to put points on the board. Special teams (punting and kicking) must create turnovers. The crowd will be noisy, but you are all professionals, and you know what you have to do. I am sick and tired of reading in the paper how great today's opponents are. Let's go out and make something happen. Now let's take a minute." With that everyone kneeled for the Lord's Prayer. I felt uncomfortable with this, so I inched my way toward the training room to hide while watching the proceedings.

Then the yelling started, "Let's go. Hit somebody out there." The game was ready to begin.

There is nothing more exciting than a professional football game. Imagine standing inside a stadium with 70,000 people yelling in the stands. You can't imagine the impact that can be felt when a linebacker hits a running back at full speed right in front of your eyes.

I remember my first game with the team. It was a home game and I was in awe of the setting. I stayed close to Dr. Rosey because I didn't know where I should be or what I would say if someone asked me who I was. After a few games, I was more comfortable standing near the players and talking to different people on the sidelines.

The one thing you must remember about being in an area of combat is that you must pay close attention to the action on the field. First, as a doctor, you should be watching the game and searching for injuries. Second, the action is so fierce that frequently plays end up out of bounds and if you are not paying attention, you can be seriously hurt.

During one game at the Orange Bowl in Miami, Dr. Rosey was more interested in locating a female friend in the stands than in watching the game. Unfortunately, there was a halfback sweep around the right end and four defensive backs tackled our player out of bounds. The next thing I knew Dr. Rosey was lying underneath the bench, twenty feet away from the sidelines. He was hurt. When he got up he was obviously in pain as he held his left shoulder. The trainer took him into the locker room and I agreed to hold down the fort on the sidelines. Yes, I was in charge, a fortuitous way to become the acting orthopedic surgeon for the team. X-rays revealed that Dr. Rosey had a fractured shoulder. He returned to the field in an arm sling with an ice bag on his shoulder.

The next six weeks were great. I got to do all the surgery with Dr. Rosey verbally assisting me. Of course he told everyone he was doing surgery, but I was holding the knife. After four to six weeks in a sling, he took it off and started to function more normally. He didn't want to be seen on national television wearing a sling. Not a good image for the team doctor.

Oh yes, national television. I will never forget the first time Dr. Rosey gave me his "T. V. Time" lecture. He didn't allow anyone except the trainer to go out on the field with him when players were hurt.

The exposure on national television was much better if only two were on the field. So I was not allowed to go.

He also said, "Never take a player off the field too quickly. Even if he's fine. Even if the player wants to leave under his own power." If the player stayed on the field, Dr. Rosey got more television exposure. True, sometimes when an injury occurred a station would break to a commercial, but other times it stayed with the game, showing the injured player for several minutes. If they were showing the injured player, they were showing Dr. Rosey.

He said, "The first thing you do when you go out onto the field before the game is to locate all of the cameras in the stadium. Learn where they are stationed." He pointed to the two across the field in the press box. These were important because they pointed right at us. "For maximum exposure the cameras should be located across the field," he reiterated. "If the cameras are in the press box behind you, all the television audience sees is your back, so the exposure for the game will be terrible. No patients will see you on T.V." He obviously had this down to a science.

He urged, "If a referee is ever injured, make sure you go out and see how he is doing, even though it's an accepted league practice that the home team doctors take care of any referee or umpire who is injured." Almost all official injuries gained excessive television coverage and Dr. Rosey insisted, "Don't be left out of these." My mentor was definitely a producer and director rolled into one.

I was lucky to have any affiliation with a professional football team, especially this one. They always came from behind to win in the last few seconds of the game and they always made the playoffs. The rewards of being with a successful professional team were more than fun. There were championship games, Super Bowls, and rings. I mean big rings. Super Bowl rings.

If you don't think the public reacts to a doctor who works with professional sports teams or has a Super Bowl ring on his finger, then you are sadly mistaken. The public is sure if you are the team orthopedist for a professional sports team, you are the best at what you do. Patients refer other patients to your office just so they can get a glimpse of your rings. They're big and sparkly and impressive. Patients like to put them on their fingers. Mothers bring in cameras and take pictures. It doesn't make any difference whether you got the job politically or any other way. You must be good. You are the team doctor. It shows how misinformed the public really is. In fact, most team physicians are chosen because they are friends of the owners or for some other nonscientific reason.

What other marketing perks are in store for team physicians? Well, any time they talk about an injured player in the newspaper the doctor's name is frequently mentioned. If a player is about to undergo surgery, the operating surgeon will almost always be quoted. Free advertising? You bet. Lots of it. Circulating to thousands of people.

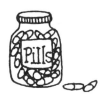

11. Tinseltown Doc

A FEW other experiences cling to my memory of this elective with Dr. Rosey. I was told I could help the office run on time if I would renew prescriptions for patients. How difficult could that be? The pharmacy would call up and want a renewal. I'd get on the phone and say, sure. No such luck.

Dr. Rosey was excessively generous about handing out medication like Percodan that required filling out a special prescription form. Often he would write twenty to thirty of these prescriptions a day, each for fifty to one hundred pills. This was strong stuff, stronger than codeine. There wasn't anything illegal about this. But I had been taught that if a patient needed pain medication this strong, he should be in the hospital. The exception was terminal cancer patients. They needed lots of this stuff and didn't need to be in a hospital to die.

I went along with this for a few weeks. I must have written at least one hundred of these prescriptions and then I had to stop. I couldn't look myself in the mirror anymore. I couldn't prescribe these addicting drugs for people with minor pain. I told Hilda I wouldn't do it anymore because it was not in the best interest of the patients. They could get by on codeine, or even Advil, which didn't require such a fuss. As you can imagine, this was another black mark Hilda held against me.

That wasn't all Dr. Rosey prescribed. He was giving athletes anabolic steroids and movies stars aphrodisiacs, like Quaalude. Did I want to be a doctor for the stars bad enough that I would compromise my ethics as a physician? What about the Hippocratic Oath? I admit I was tempted, but I didn't. I couldn't.

As my elective in Tinseltown drew toward a close, Dr. Rosey took me to dinner at an exclusive restaurant. He told me that I was the most mature resident he had ever known and I would be a great addition to his practice. He was willing to make me a partner in three years and he assured me that the money was well worth it. In addition, he could say without question, because he was a friend of the owner, I would be the heir apparent to the orthopedic job with the football team. This sounded good.

But somehow this news didn't feel quite so wonderful. It lacked the strong impact that I had felt upon getting accepted into medical school, or being accepted into the Aggie residency program. I told him how complimented I felt. I knew he was serious as he had even written a letter to my parents telling them what a nice young man I was and how proud they should be to have a son like me. I told him I was thrilled at the opportunity and would definitely consider it, but I wanted to discuss it with my wife. She had already stated on many occasions that she would never raise our children in Southern California.

The last few months were educationally very productive. I had a unique opportunity to spend a few days a week learning arthroscopy from Dr. Puff, the man who virtually invented its use in the United States. This was a new instrument that allowed the surgeon to repair many problems in the knee through three tiny holes with the use of a fiberoptic scope. This meant no more large incisions. The patient could walk the same day after surgery. Dr. Rosey was clearly not thrilled I was doing this. First of all, it meant I spent several hours out of his office, two to three times a week. Second, the doctor who invented this neat little tool was gaining international notoriety, creating envy in Dr. Rosey. But he knew I desperately wanted to learn from the best. He also knew that if I stayed around it would be a great advertisement that his new associate had trained with the big gun in arthroscopy.

People from all over the country flew into Southern California to have Dr. Puff operate on their knees. Many flew in on their own private jets and left the same day.

My working with Dr. Puff was another of those instances of being in the right place at the right time. While working in Dr. Rosey's office, I heard that a resident from the local university had contracted a serious illness and was unable to participate in the arthroscopy elective with Dr. Puff. I was the only resident available on such short notice.

The method of learning from Dr. Puff was extraordinary. He smoked at least three packs of cigarettes a day. He couldn't go longer than ten to fifteen minutes without lighting up. We would start a case together, then he would quickly state, "You can see that the medial meniscus (cartilage) looks good, but there is a small tear in the lateral meniscus. Why don't you go ahead and fix it and I'll be right back." He would return after his cigarette and either tell me I had done a good job or that one area of the cartilage could use a little more trimming. I learned quickly by this method and I learned well. By the time I left, I felt confident that with a little more practice I could be one of the best arthroscopists in the country. After all, I had learned from the Master.

I did several of Dr. Puff's cases, and by the time I left my elective, I had arthroscopically done many of Dr. Rosey's patients too. Dr. Rosey even enjoyed watching the technique. He took pride that I was working in his office. The student was teaching the professor.

What were the experiences, though, that made me decide my future? One afternoon, I was alone in the office as Dr. Rosey had gone to a car show to exhibit his antique Mercedes. Hilda was at the hairdresser's when I received a call from a famous executive producer's assistant. He said Mr. Goldberg had been running on the beach in front of his Seacliff estate and had pulled a muscle in the back of his thigh. His boss was in such pain he could hardly walk. He insisted that Dr. Rosey come to Mr. Goldberg's home immediately. I said I was covering for Dr. Rosey and it was impossible for me to go to Seacliff. "Then the limousine will bring him to your office immediately," he said. He bragged that Dr. Rosey had frequently gone to Mr. Goldberg's house in the past because of ankle sprains and backaches.

He asked, "What did you say your name was, Doctor?" I had to apologize for being Dr. Mays and explain that I was on call that afternoon. He questioned if I had ever seen this sort of injury before. The humiliation continued as the slimy attendant inquired if I had heard of Mr. Goldberg's latest movie. I admitted that I had heard of it, but had not had the time to see it. He scolded me, saying that it was one of the leading box office attractions, and that Mr. Goldberg was the executive producer of this and many other famous productions.

I searched my mind to find a way to be nice to this arrogant pip-squeak, explaining that it was probably a very minor muscle pull and if Mr. Goldberg would get off the leg for twenty-four hours and apply some ice, it might not be so painful. Then this famous movie personality and his likewise famous muscle could limp into our office tomorrow and see Dr. Rosey.

"I don't think you understand," he replied. "Mr. Goldberg is in severe pain and needs to be cured now." I told him once again there was absolutely no way I could go to Seacliff since I had to make hospital rounds and stay close to cover the practice. But I agreed to see them in the office in about an hour if this severely injured celebrity could somehow load his fat ass into the limousine and come to Rodeo Hills. He consented.

About two hours later I was still waiting. I was slightly annoyed at myself for ruining an opportunity to go to a real movie star's home, but I just couldn't lower myself to be manipulated. Finally the entourage appeared through the back door.

Most of the important people came through the back door at Hilda's request so they wouldn't have to be seen or bothered by the common folks in the waiting room. Hilda personally put them in a room. She made a point of being around the important patients so she could log in another favor. It seemed that Mr. Goldberg was also the executive producer of many rock concerts, and Hilda claimed to get front row seats for each and every show.

I forgot to tell Hilda they had called until the last minute. She was impressed that I was able to get them to come to see me. She explained that as many times as Dr. Rosey had tried to get them to come into the office, he had always ended up travelling to Seacliff. I told her I was surprised to hear that.

I entered the room and Hilda introduced me as Dr. Rosey's associate. As she spoke, I peered over at the little wimp who had obviously spoken to me on the phone. He was four feet tall and weighed about eighty pounds. He had a washed-out appearance. In his hand was a cute little brown purse. He stared at me as if I had just put one over on him. And I had.

I couldn't believe all the gold jewelry Mr. Goldberg wore. Hilda excused herself and I asked him to remove his pants so I could see this very serious bit of orthopedic pathology. There was slight soreness on the back of the thigh. Mr. Goldberg had obviously pulled his hamstring muscle. It wasn't torn, just stretched a little. It has happened to most of us over the years a few times. "Well, Mr. Goldberg, it's just as I told your friend over the telephone. You pulled your hamstring muscle. It's just a slight sprain. I'll tape it for you today, give you some pain pills and some crutches and in a few weeks you'll be as good as new." He gave me a blank look.

"Perhaps you don't understand, Doctor. I'm sorry, what did you say your name was?" I told him. "Right," he apologized. "I have to be in the studio tomorrow for rehearsal, so I can't use crutches for two weeks. Trust me. Whatever it takes, just go ahead and fix my leg. Believe me, I can afford it. How much will it cost to fix this problem?" he begged.

I was speechless. He really didn't comprehend. This couldn't be taken care of with money. He couldn't buy a new hamstring muscle. I replied, "I'm sorry I can't just snap my fingers and make you well. If I could, I would do it for free."

"This may be funny to you, Doctor, but I don't think it's funny at all," he said angrily. I taped his thigh while his little companion stared at me as if he wanted to slit my throat. I told Mr. Goldberg as he struggled to the door with his crutches that Dr. Rosey would be back tomorrow and he could see him then. The patient felt that he could talk Dr. Rosey into coming to Seacliff tomorrow and requested that I have him call immediately upon his return.

I saw Dr. Rosey on rounds the next morning and told him of my encounter with Mr. Goldberg. He laughed and admitted he had been to the Seacliff estate a few times. "You really should have made a house call, Doc," he joked. "His house is incredible." I was afraid he would say something like that.

I told him I just didn't think it would be in the best interest of the practice for me to be gone that long, especially if another patient had a real problem and I was needed in the office quickly. He insinuated that a doctor for the stars sometimes had to go the extra mile (no pun intended) to please a celebrity, if you were to have a successful practice. I knew then that I would never return to Tinseltown. They could give me cars. They could give me gold. They could give me limousines. They could give me fame. They could keep it, all to themselves.

As the time drew near to leave, I reflected on my experience. It had been one of the greatest things that had ever happened to me. My little family and I had been able to live on the beach for six months and listen to the ocean as we dozed off to sleep. I had acquired tremendous firsthand experience in surgical techniques no other resident in my program would ever see. I had spent time with the most famous arthroscopic surgeon in the country and this would, no doubt, look very impressive on my resume. I had tasted a fascinating piece of private practice and actually rubbed elbows with many movie stars and professional athletes that I had watched for years. In addition, I had examined the knee of my favorite television cop and the most handsome cowboy of all time. I had treated the shoulder of the greatest songbird ever to sing.

The football experience was the closest to my heart. I would miss this, almost tearfully. I had become a part of the team. People knew my name and actually spoke to me. They placed my name on a seat of each charter we flew to the games. My name was on the hotel room list for all the games. And yes, the team sent me the same Christmas gift they sent Dr. Rosey, a portable television with my name inscribed on it. Feeling a part of the team was important to me. I was sad to leave.

Dr. Rosey and I had one last supper at his home, and this was one of the few times I ever saw his wife. Their home was modest but in a very affluent area. They had a pool and a maid.

Before dinner he showed me his VCR room with walls of tapes he had stored over the past fifteen years. He had taped every football game the team had played on national television since he had become their physician. He would come home the day after the game to watch himself. He showed me a tape of a game they had played the year before in Denver, when it snowed. He had had to put on a large team jacket so he wouldn't freeze to death. When one of the offensive guards was injured, you couldn't even recognize Dr. Rosey as he ran onto the field. He was annoyed. His exposure was poor.

I was embarrassed because as we sat at the table to eat, his wife kept ringing a bell for the black maid. I felt like I was in the Deep

South. I was very uncomfortable. But I took the initiative to make a toast to him and what he had meant to me personally and professionally over the past six months. The experience had helped me grow as a person. This had been an opportunity that was far beyond my expectations. In spite of the weird people and all of the rah-rah, I was very lucky to have met him. I assured him that I would give his offer serious consideration. My wife kicked my shin under the table.

The following day I sadly said good-bye. Dr. Rosey had been my mentor and my friend. I had admired what he had accomplished over the years and I felt a real void about to begin in my life. I knew I would especially miss all of his secretaries, who had been wonderful to me. But I wouldn't miss Hilda at all. She was, in fact, the single biggest reason I knew I could never return to this practice. She ruled the roost and I couldn't handle that. I had found out over the last six months that his practice had had five doctors come and go over the past three years. At one point or another I had touched base with all of them in the hospital. It was obvious Hilda was the main reason they had each left the practice. She was brash and rude. And she cared only about Dr. Rosey's fame and his celebrity patients.

Dr. Rosey had spent six months being the professor he had always wanted to be. He told me as I parted, as a last-ditch effort to lure me toward the practice, that he would be honored if he could leave his practice to me one day. He hoped that during my fourth year of residency I could find the time to come to the football games. He would be happy to arrange this for me. "Yes, I'd like that," I said.

We actually embraced as I left. I told him he had been like a father to me. He had spent time with me. He had been my pal. I had spent more time on the sidelines and in airplanes with this guy for the past six months than I had ever spent with my father.

Finally, I went to thank Hilda. She was pleasant, but I could see she was worried. She knew Dr. Rosey liked me and wanted me to be a partner. I fantasized that she saw her reign coming to an end. The practice would take on a different direction if I returned. She gave me a parting peck on the cheek and told me to contact her if she could ever do anything for me. I never saw her again.

I left through the back door, just like the stars. Before leaving the parking lot I gave the attendant a bottle of wine, as he had frequently parked my car when I was in a hurry.

As I drove to the beach to pick up my family, I felt good about the job I had done. I had worked diligently over the past six months, and even though the practice had given an enormous amount to me, I had given an enormous amount in return. I had dictated hundreds of histories and physicals, operative reports, and discharge summaries for Dr. Rosey, not to mention the numerous orders and chart notes. I knew much of what I had done had been only busywork, but after all, that was part of my verbal contract. I felt as though most of his patients liked me and many were sorry to hear I was leaving. I had the feeling that somehow this experience had set the stage for me and that greater things would come. I was on my way.

I must admit I was depressed as we headed down the freeway. It was a real letdown. I knew I was leaving one of the greatest encounters of my life, only to return to being a lowly resident. At least I was about to enter my fourth year. I would be the chief resident in charge of the junior residents, the interns, and the medical students. I would only have to answer to the faculty. And I would have to begin thinking about what I would do with the rest of my life. Where would I go? With whom would I practice? How would I make this monumental decision? Who would help me make it? During the ride home, many times I thought of turning around to be with Dr. Rosey.

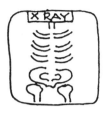

12. Return to Residency

ONCE at the residency I realized how good my training had been compared to the other fourth-year residents. Not that I was better than anybody else, but I knew what I was doing. I was comfortable in the middle of the night handling almost any orthopedic emergency.

I felt good that many people were supportive of my leave and were impressed that I had become somewhat famous around the university. Many had seen me on television and I began to understand how Dr. Rosey felt.

But there were lots of negatives to my return, too. The start of my fourth year meant that I would be out in a year and I had better start thinking about where to practice my trade for the rest of my life. I knew I didn't want to be in Southern California, but I didn't want anyone else to know that. I was always taught to keep all my options open.

Other negatives included the fact that the chief resident had to work hand in hand with the faculty. They were too important to spend much time with the junior residents or students. The faculty operated only with the chief resident.

So why was this so bad? Dr. Bugg, the new faculty person on my first rotation, was an absolute prick. It was torture. One resident prior to me said he was the most peculiar human being he had ever met. He was a hand surgeon who had recently joined the faculty after his training in New Orleans. He had come to the university for only one reason. It was a stepping stone to private practice. He was there to steal cases from the residents so he could go out and make it on his own. This meant that, as chief resident, I lost the opportunity to sur-gically handle major cases. I didn't mind this because I had spent a lot of time in my third year with Dr. Buttons, who was a noted hand surgeon and could run circles around Dr. Bugg anytime. But I still had to put up with his incredible nonsense for four months, and I didn't know if I could take it.

How peculiar was this guy? First, he didn't allow any talking dur-ing surgery because it cut down on his concentration and increased the chance of infection. Of course there had never been any scientific study to prove this stupid claim, but he was the boss. You can imagine how fruitful it was to try to learn an intricate subject like hand surgery without the professor talking or demonstrating during surgery. We needed to hear things like, "Here you see the flexor muscle where it crosses over the nerve." Or, "Notice the pulley for this tendon stops here." He allowed none of that.

My first encounter with Dr. Bugg was after he had done several cases one day. After the first case, none of the students came to observe. He asked me where everyone had gone. I told him as diplo-matically as I could that they had a lot of work to do on the orthopedic ward and they weren't learning anything here because no one was talking to them. He lectured that you can learn by watch-ing. I explained that the incisions were so small that the students couldn't see from behind the table and he wouldn't allow them to scrub so they could get closer. He shook his head and walked away.

I saw Dr. Buttons in conference later that day and I told him about my confrontation with Dr. Bugg. He totally agreed with me but asked me nicely to pick one student to attend each surgery so Dr. Bugg could feel like a professor. After all, Dr. Bugg was the new fac-ulty member and we wanted to make him feel needed. Sure thing. I agreed to do this because I liked Dr. Buttons, and I told the students to decide among themselves each surgery day who would suffer.

Those four months were hell. I hated Dr. Bugg and he hated me. I must admit I antagonized him any time I could. "It's interesting that you do this particular tendon transfer, since I noticed that Dr. Buttons uses the flexor carpi ulnaris," I jabbed. He told me that there were several acceptable procedures. Of course I knew that but I was just doing my best to irritate him.

The nurses despised him too. In surgery, he wouldn't let them talk either. When they did, he held his hand up as if to say, shut up. He would simply point to the instrument he wanted. This didn't happen often, though, because he had his own, self-made apron which he wore on his chest to hold all of his tools. He looked like someone in a space suit. If only we could have launched him back to the unfortunate planet from which he had escaped. Or had they blasted him away?

The other weak link in the faculty was the pediatric orthopedic service professor, Dr. Rail. He was Mr. Cool with the students because he loved to joke around. But with the residents he felt the need to constantly harass us. He seemed to be saying, "I know more than you do and I always will." He loved to read a totally irrelevant article and then question us about it the next day. Why didn't we know that?

He didn't like me because I knew so much more about operating on the knee and shoulder than he, thanks to Dr. Rosey. I had published an article on pectoralis tears of the shoulder while I was with Dr. Rosey and he told me what was wrong with the article. Once I asked him how many pectoralis tears he had seen. He said, "A bunch." I'm quite certain he had never seen one. I asked him how many he had ever operated on. He said, "A few." He was a liar, but the professor had to lie to sound like a professor. If these professors could have operated at all or gotten along with people, they would have been in the community practicing orthopedics.

It also bothered him that I got over five hundred reprint requests for the publication. He had published a bunch of nothing articles in the past and requests for reprints were few and far between, according to his personal secretary, who also hated him. He was furious when I asked him what was the best way to order more reprints of my article. I told him the five hundred I had received gratis with my publication were all gone.

He did know something about hip surgery, though. He was experienced in total joint surgery, but he contradicted many of the things that Dr. Smooth had taught us, so I needed to retrain myself to do it Dr. Rail's way. I did it to a certain extent, just to make peace. His way was definitely not better.

13. Ski Doc

ANOTHER interesting chore I was given as chief resident was to organize a sports medicine elective at a nearby ski resort for students rotating on the orthopedic surgery service. It was Dr. Smooth who had dreamed up this idea before he left. It was actually a good idea but was never well developed.

The plan was to place a resident or faculty member at a ski resort for one week at a time. The faculty person would be in charge of the first aid station. There was a full-time nurse employed by the ski resort who remained in the clinic at all times. If she needed the doctor, she would beep him on the slopes. It was called a sports medicine ski elective at the medical school because the students could sign up and spend two weeks at the resort. They were required to stay in the clinic with the nurse, who would teach them basic first aid.

In return for donating a week's service, the doctor would get free ski lift passes for himself and his family and the use of a condominium for that week. Sound good, so far? Actually, most of the time it was. But the organization was a nightmare.

The entire faculty at the university wanted to go ski for a week. The word spread around the medical school that you could sign up for a week and get free lift passes and a condominium. Pediatricians, heart surgeons, and psychiatrists all inquired. This raised a question. Should you be able to act as the doctor for a week if you knew nothing about orthopedic surgery? Let's face it. Ninety-five percent of injuries that occurred on the ski slopes were broken bones, dislocations, etc. So you can imagine the politics I had to deal with.

There were about twenty-five weeks in a ski season. Of course the orthopedic professors preferred certain ones such as Christmas, New Year's, and Washington's birthday because they didn't have to take their children out of school. I just laughed and gave them those choice times. Why? Because these were, by far, the busiest times at a ski resort, when the first aid clinic was usually full of injured patients. The person on duty seldom had much time to ski. Essentially, they went away for a week in the snow, but had to work much harder than expected.

Our resident nurse at the resort gave me a hassle when I sent up a heart surgeon. She knew this was going to be a bad week on the first day when a young skier came in bragging how he had just made a great jump off a hill but had landed inappropriately on his chest. He complained of severe pain from an obvious chest bruise and the heart surgeon examined him and asked if he had any history of aortic valve stenosis. The frightened patient grabbed his shirt and ran out the door bare-chested. The "cardiac kid" asked the nurse if he had said something wrong.

This poor guy didn't know how to put on a splint. There was no way he could relocate a dislocated shoulder. Why did I send this guy? I explained he was a close friend of one of the orthopedic professors and I had been asked nicely to give him a week. She told me that after his first day, she didn't even bother to beep him the rest of the week. Together with the student, she splinted all the fractures and sewed up all the lacerations. They manned the clinic without this heart surgeon, out of fear of what he might do if given a chance.

I finally went up for a week to console the nurse and to do my one-week stint. I picked a time that wouldn't be crowded so I could get to know the operation and take inventory. The first aid station was stocked with a lot of supplies, including drugs, which had to be monitored. But my week wasn't peaceful.

The first day I decided to take a few runs, so I grabbed the beeper and wished the nurse farewell. About an hour later I was paged. At the top of the mountain I asked the operator to call the clinic to see what was happening. She told me that the nurse needed me immediately, as a patient with a severe scalp laceration was bleeding profusely.

I headed down the hill as fast as possible. I was not an expert skier, but I moved swiftly. Some suggested my form resembled a runaway freight train. Even at a fast pace it took ten minutes to get down the hill.

While paralleling down the slope, I realized I knew little about scalp lacerations. In fact, I knew nothing other than that the scalp had a very good blood supply, so most cuts healed quickly. I would just suture it up. When I arrived I stepped out of my skis and walked through the lodge toward the clinic's front door so I could warm up my hands. The woman and daughter sitting in the waiting room looked petrified. The lady had large blood stains all over her bright blue ski outfit.

As I entered the exam room the nurse gave me a very blank look. This was unusual for her, after the compound fractures and punctured eyeballs she had seen. The patient was lying on the table and he looked pale. "Hi, I'm Dr. Mays," I said. "Sorry to keep you waiting, but I got down the hill as fast as I could and that's not too fast." He chuckled but the nurse didn't.

"Mr. Jackson fell down and cut his scalp on the edge of his ski," the nurse uttered. When I asked her to remove the big compression bandage that she had placed on his head, she motioned her eyes upward. She suggested I put on some sterile gloves while she removed the dressing. Oh my God! This was so gross even I became light-headed. This man had been scalped. His entire scalp was turned back behind his head and was hanging down behind his neck. I'd never seen anything like this. "How does it look, Doc?" he asked. I couldn't believe my eyes. I didn't know what to say. "Well, you have a large cut on the front of your forehead," I remarked. What the hell was I going to do?

I knew one thing, I couldn't manage this injury. This was, at the very least, a plastic surgery case. I instructed the nurse to cover up this mess, and I told the patient that this would best be done in surgery. I would send him over to the local hospital about one hour away. But the nurse remarked, "Unfortunately, Doctor, the roads are all closed in both directions due to the heavy snowstorm." Oh, no, I have to call a friend of mine at the university who is a plastic surgeon and ask him what the hell to do.

It figured. Both he and his associate were away at a meeting, probably basking in the sun, and here I was freezing with this unsolvable problem. I signaled for the nurse to come around the corner so we could huddle. "What do you think we should do?" I pleaded. She reminded me he was bleeding. Well, when the going gets tough, the tough get going. I went back and invited the wife to come into the exam room as the nurse talked with the daughter.

I explained our dilemma in detail to these folks. The laceration was severe, the roads were closed, he was bleeding, and I was just a bone doctor. As often is the case, they asked what I suggested. I explained that the scalp had a very good blood supply and if we copiously washed the entire scalp wound and sewed the thing up, the laceration would heal, hopefully.

I explained I couldn't guarantee the results but that was the best idea I had. I didn't want this guy to bleed to death. They agreed. The wife wished me good luck, kissed him good-bye, and retreated to the waiting room. Neither she nor the patient looked very confident.

I told the nurse what I had in mind. "You're kidding, of course," she said. She told me I was crazy and went off shaking her head. We got out a sterile tray, plenty of sutures, and I irrigated the hell out of the wound. I remembered from medical school, "The solution to pollution is dilution." The scalp was still severely bleeding but I felt this was a good sign for healing. We prepped the scalp sterilely and injected it with loads of novocaine. I sewed and the nurse cut the sutures.

The medical student sat and watched in shock. The nurse was angry at me for attempting this feat, but I didn't know what else to do. When we were done, I put several drains in his scalp for the blood to exit over the next several hours. It actually looked quite good. But who knew what would happen down the road? The student helped me wrap the scalp with a large compression dressing that made the patient look like he was wearing a bicycle helmet. We gave him a shot of intramuscular antibiotics in his thigh and he walked out under his own power.

Since they were staying close to my condominium, I asked if I could stop by in a few hours and check the dressing. That impressed them. The nauseated medical staff cleaned up the bloody room and we took care of several smaller injuries before the day ended. We adjourned to the bar to talk about this incredible scalp injury.

While we were sitting in the bar, a waitress came to get the nurse.

The cook had cut his finger. He was at the first aid station with ice on it. We put down our drinks and followed her. The cut wasn't bad but rather deep in one area, where it just missed the digital nerve that goes out to the fingertip. Here we go again. We prepped and draped the finger and sewed up the wound. I let the student do most of the work, since the draping prevented the cook from seeing who was doing what.

This turned out to be a very worthwhile case. Not because it was interesting, but because the cook was an important person to know at a ski resort. The next day he noticed me sitting outside on the deck at lunchtime and asked if I'd eaten yet. I told him I was about to go and stand in line. He told the nurse and me to sit tight, grab a table, and he'd be right back. The clinic was quiet, so it was perfect timing. We left the student in charge and this, of course, made her happy and proud.

You can see why I could never be a professor. I was too nice to the student. I told her that I would man the clinic after lunch so she would get a chance to ski. The nurse said that was a first. We sat basking in the sun waiting for lunch. The cook returned, finger bandaged and all, carrying a large plate stacked high with beef ribs, French fries, and two large glasses of beer. "Thanks again for your help, yesterday." I'm happy to report that this took place every day at lunch for the entire week. We worked hard but we played hard.

The weather became colder, and for me skiing needs to be done while I can still feel my fingertips. When it turns too cold or it snows so hard I can't see, I head for the lodge and have a hot toddy.

The day after the scalping, I was in the clinic examining a broken thumb when the nurse received a phone call from the ski patrol that a man had collapsed on the slopes. They thought he was unconscious and they were bringing him down immediately. He arrived on a stretcher ten minutes later with at least seven ski patrol personnel. I didn't like the looks of this at all.

As the team hurled him onto the examination table, I judged his age to be about forty. His face was blue, he was motionless, and there was no heartbeat. I started resuscitation efforts immediately with the help of the medical student and the nurse. I thought the man was dead on arrival, since he had no pulse and no spontaneous respirations, but I felt we had to try. I was uncomfortable pronouncing any human being dead. I was just a bone setter. I didn't do that sort of thing. To make matters worse, his wife came in, said she was a nurse and would be willing to help. But I told her I thought it was best for her to stay in the waiting room.

I yelled for someone to get the intubation kit so I could put a tube down his throat to assist his breathing, as we were not having much luck oxygenating him. I did this successfully and I quietly thanked the brief anesthesiology rotation that had taught me how to do this. I also started a quick intravenous line for fluids. But we didn't seem to be making much progress. Although he was pinking up a bit, he still had only a faint pulse. I pounded once on his chest to see if I could start a spontaneous heartbeat, and when this didn't work, I tried once more. In frustration, I had the nurse call for a nearby helicopter service to get this poor guy over to the hospital. I still believed all along he was dead. About five minutes had passed since he had gotten to the clinic. Nothing was working. Resuscitation efforts were continued by the nurse and the student as I frantically tried to figure out what to do next. We had no means to shock him.

The CPR continued until a helicopter showed up, about fifteen minutes later. This was a small chopper that was going to make CPR very difficult on the way to the hospital. There was a small area for the stretcher in the back seat but not enough room for the nurse and me. I had to lean into the back from the front seat while the two of us continued this obviously futile effort as the helicopter flew precariously over the mountaintops.

He was pronounced dead on arrival. I felt horrible. I was a fish out of water. I didn't sign up for this. I came up for a week to do a little skiing and already I had seen two terrible non-orthopedic injuries that I was not qualified to treat. Or was I? After all, I was an M.D. I sat around sulking in the emergency room lounge, talking with the emergency room doctor while the helicopter people did their paperwork. The nurse called back to the clinic and learned the man's wife was on her way to the hospital.

I reviewed our resuscitation efforts in detail with the emergency room doctor. He assured me we had done all of the right things. He agreed with me that the man was probably dead on the slope after suffering a massive heart attack. I wasn't asking because I was afraid we would be sued but rather to see if other things should have been tried, in case this ever happened to me again. I asked him if I should have injected some medicine directly into the heart and he said no. We had nothing else to do. We had no defibrillator paddles.

When I returned home I reviewed this case with the university attorneys as to whether we should have had more equipment to deal with this type of catastrophe. After some discussion it was agreed by all that our clinic was merely a first aid station to treat injuries temporarily until more comprehensive care could be obtained. Emergency room experts and attorneys both commented that if more fancy equipment was obtained, the clinic and the university would essentially have to assure the public that the medical staff present was properly trained to use it. And besides, if we got a defibrillator, why not have an EKG machine, an x-ray unit, and a laboratory? Where do you stop? Where do you draw the line? They had a very good point.

The remainder of my week was eventful but less stressful. The medical student thought this was the greatest elective she had ever signed up for. She said, "This place is definitely where the action is." I was glad someone was happy. I knew the nurse and I had been much less excited about the events so far. We were emotionally drained.

Toward the end of the week we saw two people within three hours who had dislocated their shoulders. Skiers got their poles caught in trees and ripped their shoulders out of the sockets. I let the medical student reduce both of these, and her face was something to behold when she felt her first humeral head clunk back into the socket. She was "jazzed." She was learning a lot about sports medicine and the injuries and treatments associated with it.

As always in medicine, there was an amusing side. One afternoon I was in the clinic throwing away outdated drugs when a lady came in but refused to discuss her problem with the nurse. She demanded to speak with the doctor immediately. I figured the nurse was getting annoyed, so I went out front and told the lady to step "into my office." She was stunning but appeared frightened. I introduced myself and asked how I could help. She stated she had fallen forward on her skis and was concerned that she had ruptured her left breast implant. I was shocked. I wanted to laugh but caught myself as she seemed "dead" serious. I was searching for something intelligent to say.

"What makes you think it's busted?" I smirked. "I felt a pop," she answered.

I took a further history from the patient and learned she had had bilateral breast implants done a year ago in San Diego. I finally came up with an idea which I felt would satisfy us both. I suggested I take a look. I'm not a complete idiot though, so I asked the patient's permission for the nurse to join us. She consented, reluctantly. I gave her a gown and retreated to the front lobby to regain my composure.

On examination both breasts appeared wonderful to me. They were both perfect in size and shape. In fact, they were terrific. Anyway, I told her I didn't "feel" anything that would make me suspicious of a rupture. Of course I had never seen a ruptured breast implant. I further speculated that there was no inflammation around the breast tissue suggesting irritation by silicone or other foreign substances. I was damn impressed with my reasoning. But she still appeared worried. So I offered to call her plastic surgeon in San Diego and I thought it best that she return the next day for another check. The nurse gave me a very dirty look.

My final day in the clinic was the best. The sun came out and I took a few early-morning runs down the slopes. I returned at 10:00 a.m. to conduct my own private clinic. I first unveiled my patient's scalp dressing and looked at the wound. I was nervous, as the night before I had spoken with the plastic surgeon in San Diego. After I had asked about the lady with the breast problem, I told him about my predicament with the scalp laceration. He thought I had done the right thing to control bleeding but admitted he had had a similar patient in the military and the entire flap had sloughed. That made me feel uncomfortable all night long as I tried to get to sleep unsuccessfully. But today the flap looked good. There was a small amount of bloody drainage, but the skin looked healthy so far. The nurse and student redressed the wound, and I wished the patient well and pleaded with him to give me some follow-up in a few weeks. I handed him my card. I knew if I didn't hear from him I would hear from his attorney. He thanked me profusely and his wife handed me a bottle of white wine.

My next patient arrived to have her breast checked. She looked better today but still acted concerned. I didn't want to tell her that I had talked to the plastic surgeon, who had reassured me nothing was wrong and that this patient was a chronic worry wart. I felt it was in my best interest to take one more look. They looked wonderful again and felt good, too. Hey, I was entitled to this. I had had a hard week. Both the medical student and the nurse made me buy them lunch while they sat there and questioned my medical indications for a second examination of this breast in less than twenty-four hours. I told them I was trying to set an example of what a caring, thorough physician should be like. I told them I objected strenuously to their suggestion that I was turned on, but my two comrades ordered yet another round of drinks on me as punishment.

14. The Professor

THE CHIEF residency was also the time to taste the professorial role. I led a team of junior residents, interns, and medical students on rounds every day and was in charge of the clinics, unless a faculty member was there. I did a fair amount of teaching and this was fun because I always enjoyed it.

I was never in favor of making students look bad, so I could never have made a good professor. I preferred to teach to learn. I'd ask a question and if no one knew the answer, I gave it and explained it. I didn't believe in making anyone feel bad. I think all of my students left the orthopedic service with a lot of essential knowledge. If they picked up a few pearls, that was good enough for me, like knowing the severe fractures from the simple ones, knowing good surgical technique, and knowing when to cast and when to splint. It would be these types of principles that would help them later in their careers, no matter what specialty they pursued.

Later I became even more of a professor. The article I had written when I was with Dr. Rosey, on pectoralis tears of the shoulder, was one of the first to be published on the subject. It drew international attention and I was asked to present the paper at many conferences across the country. It was fun to travel at the university's expense. Dr. Buttons was delighted because it made him and the department look good. He loved seeing my name on various scientific programs, which created a positive reflection on him.

The first meeting was at the American College of Sports Medicine in Hawaii. This was a well-attended meeting, and even Dr. Rosey came to watch me. He was proud because his name was on the article too. To show my appreciation, I made him my discussant for the paper. I was afraid for him, as this wasn't his forte. He probably had not been in front of a real audience since his bar mitzvah. All his television exposure would do him no good here. But he did all right and fortunately I had answered most of the questions already.

My next meeting was more memorable. I went to Gainesville, Florida to present the paper. I tried to sidestep this trip but a friend of Dr. Buttons from Gainesville called and persuaded me to attend. My surgery schedule was so full, I took the midnight flight to Miami. I didn't sleep a wink because I was seated next to a beautiful young attorney who had just passed the bar exam. She worked in a district attorney's office. She had some fascinating stories to tell and a great pair of legs. She loved doctors, as her father was one.

I transferred in Miami to Gainesville and arrived about 9:00 a.m. for an 11:00 a.m. lecture. I found the lecture hall and was excited that my name was on a large poster outside the room. It was a beautiful day in Florida, so I strolled outside the lecture hall and parked myself under a tree on a large grassy area. These university settings were beautiful and I enjoyed watching the co-eds play frisbee. Then I committed the ultimate sin. I fell sound asleep. Here I was, over three thousand miles away from home at the university's expense, about to sleep through a lecture I was suppose to present. And no one even knew I was there.

Luckily a frisbee hit me in the head. I jumped up, stunned. Where was I? Oh my God! What time was it? I grabbed my watch, and saw it was ten minutes to eleven. Oh no! I quickly brushed off the grass from my pants and shirt, grabbed my briefcase, and ran in to the room. A throng of people watched as I walked down the side aisle toward the stage. I still felt half-asleep, but this was how I had given some of my best lectures. A gray-haired man was at the podium explaining the day's program, and then he began apologizing for me, saying that I had a long way to travel and he hoped I would be there soon. Then he spotted me and started to giggle. I'm sure I looked like hell and didn't smell much better, as I had perspired a lot while sleeping in the sun.

But the lecture went off beautifully. The audience seemed pleased during the question-and-answer session. Afterwards a faculty member invited me to lunch with the residents. He implied that the residents in Florida couldn't compare to the California crop. They needed to write papers to promote the university. I wished Dr. Buttons could hear this. One of the residents drove me to the airport and I was back home in twenty-four hours. I didn't have a great deal of fun, but it was hard to be a professor.

My last exposure as a professor was running a medical education seminar for the university. The department of postgraduate medicine was made up of several incompetents, but one older lady was the exception. She decided the university could profit by offering a sports medicine seminar and have yours truly be the main attraction because of my recent football affiliation. I was approached with an offer to chair the course, which we decided to hold in Bayview. Success or failure, I would get paid. And it would look good on my resume.

The budget for the course was based on fifty participants so we wouldn't look bad the first year. I had some say about the faculty on the program, but the university insisted on having the last word for political reasons. Some real deadbeat professors came and gave their usual canned talks. Luckily, ninety people signed up and the course was a big success. I was given much of the credit because I gave several talks and marketed the course. I was asked to do it again the next year, and this was the start of an extra career for me.

There was some dissension my senior year. Dr. Buttons, our chief, decided to step down as orthopedic chairman and a young aggressive man from a nearby county hospital was hired to take over. I didn't care because I was close to leaving. But this fellow brought along an entirely new philosophy to surgery. Dr. Bottoms had taught us that if you can treat something conservatively, don't operate. Surgery brought complications which ultimately brought grief. But this new chief, Dr. Fixation, operated on everything. If it was broken, he'd fix it, plate it, rod it, or screw it. I'm not saying this was always wrong, but it was totally different from what I had been taught for three years.

People who had broken thigh bones no longer lay in traction for six weeks. We rodded them and they walked the next day. They were out of the hospital a few days later. Making rounds on the same patient daily for six weeks got old fast. The newer residents loved Dr. Fixation, as they could see they were going to do a lot of surgery.

But this guy fixed a lot of fractures that didn't need fixing. He had no fear. He left plates sticking out of wounds. Infections didn't bother him. The rest of us couldn't sleep, but he just kept cutting. His surgical indications were marginal. But he was chief, so we kept quiet.

Poor Dr. Buttons stayed on the faculty part-time and had to sit in x-ray conference every week and see all these cases, after he had spent a lifetime trying to teach residents not to operate unless it was necessary. He was never asked for his opinion, although he clearly had the most wisdom in the room. His nervousness was particularly funny as he would sit in his chair and viciously pull up his socks. There was one conference when Dr. Fixation showed a shoulder fracture which had been fixed with about thirty screws. Dr. Buttons responded by pulling his ankle-high socks up to his groin.

My main objective now was to figure out where I would hang my shingle after residency. As you can imagine, there was no shortage of suggestions. I was invited to join the staff at the local prepaid health plan and this appealed to me for one reason. Although the salary was not great, I could do all the arthroscopy I wanted, thus improving my skills without politicking for referrals.

There were also two offers from local orthopedists. One man was very quiet but had a large sports medicine practice. His office was small and he was very tight. The second offer was from Dr. Round, who heavily recruited me. He said I could start off by working for him while he went on vacation and he would pay me half of what I billed. This sounded the best, as I was hearing some unfavorable comments about the other doctor. I went with Dr. Round.

During the last month of my final year, the faculty wished me luck and reassured me that I would do well. I received lots of advice about how to get started and develop a practice. It was repeatedly suggested that I introduce myself to all the emergency room doctors for referrals. Yes, I would have to accept some patients with no insurance, but I would get some good cases too, like little old ladies with broken hips.

I applied for privileges at two local hospitals and had no problems being credentialed. One hospital was highly reputable and run by the Sisters. The other was less reputable because of a recent scandal that had attracted national attention. It seemed that an anesthesiologist had orally copulated women behind the sheets while they were under anesthesia for surgery. This went on for several months. Even though some staff nurses knew of this and reported it to their supervisors, it was covered up. This sad doctor was sent to a prison for mentally disturbed sex offenders and only a few hands were slapped. But the hundreds of women who reviewed their hospital bills and saw that this anesthesiologist had treated them were delirious. Lawsuits were filed by the dozens. The whole thing left a bad taste in everyone's mouth.

Dr. Cataract, the chief of the orthopedic section at this same hospital, was equally unimpressive. He had also graduated from Aggie University but it was a well-known fact at the medical school that the faculty was ashamed of Dr. Cataract. In fact, he was the worst resident they had ever trained. He wore fancy clothes and drove expensive cars. When he interviewed me, he warned me not to become too busy too soon. He made no reference to the fact that we had trained at the same facility and he seemed annoyed that I was coming to the community.

I was hoping the rest of the community wasn't like Dr. Cataract. It was obvious that he didn't want me around. At least he could have been friendlier. He could have wished me luck and welcomed me. But I knew what I had to do over the next year. I needed to introduce myself to everyone in the area, let them know I was available, and let them see that I could do good work.

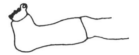

15. First Year Out

MY FIRST DAY out in the real world started with a pep talk from Dr. Round. I would be covering his practice while he vacationed for a month. He was the busiest partner in a group of four. Dr. Heel was primarily a foot doctor, and Dr. Law practiced legal medicine. Dr. Mouse was a young orthopedist who had graduated from Aggie University two years before me. Dr. Round told me I couldn't expect to be busy for several months, but his practice would allow me to get started, and he wished me luck. He reiterated that I would earn fifty percent of my gross receipts and I shouldn't worry about the money my first year. He told me I was young and money wasn't that necessary yet. It was reassuring to know I could make my house payments with plaster of paris.

I went to both emergency rooms in town the first day. I wanted to introduce myself to the doctors and begin playing the game. These were important players in my life because I felt if the emergency room doctors and nurses liked me, they would call me. I gave my usual spiel that I was just starting out, had no patients, was hungry, and would take any cases they had, good or bad. I promised to respond quickly, which the nurses said was unlike most other orthopedists in town. I went to the coffee room every morning for a doughnut and to the lunch room at noontime to mingle with my medical colleagues.

The first few days were fun. It was a new experience to be a boy again. "Yes, sir" and "No, sir." I ran into Dr. Airhead my second day. I had to be nice to this bozo because he was a friend of my parents. I don't think they cared that much for him but he owned a home at nearby Lake Nevada and he gave them his cabin every summer for a couple of weeks.

He was also the guy who took care of my broken leg when I was a little boy. I remember this vividly because he cut the cast off my leg without telling me about the noisy cast saw. He merely grabbed my leg and started sawing. I was petrified. I told my dad, who apologized for his poor bedside manner. Apparently he was notorious for this at the hospital.

He had unacceptable hours for making rounds on his hospital patients and routinely visited them between ten and eleven o'clock at night. That was not an indication of a doctor who was organized.

He practiced with Dr. Finicky, who had a decent reputation but was a well-known nitpicker. He ran around the hospital like a little rat. I had worked with him extensively at the local student health service while I was a resident, and he turned out to be a marginal orthopedist. He would not operate on someone unless the indications were stabbing him in the chest. He would see a young athlete injured in an intramural football game who had twisted a knee which then locked up three to four times. For teaching purposes, he told the residents the differential diagnosis could be inflammation, tumor, loose body, or maybe a torn cartilage. The kid obviously had a torn cartilage and was begging for surgery, now. But Dr. Finicky had to play the professorial role and try to teach non-operative treatment. All the residents dreaded his clinics because they got to do very little surgery.

The days began to get interesting. My availability in the emergency rooms was paying off. I would get at least two to three calls a day. The emergency room docs were great. They told me that if I came at all hours of the day and night for the bad cases, then they would call me for the good ones, too. If I had to clean out a few legs that had compound fractures from motorcycle accidents, I would also get my share of little old ladies with broken hips. None of the local orthopedists wanted to assist me in surgery during the late hours. But I was told there were lots of older general surgeons in the community who would love to assist, day or night.

I became busy in a hurry, much busier than Dr. Round had expected. And with my own cases. I fulfilled my obligation to him and took good care of his uninteresting patients. He stopped by every week to see how I was doing and to issue me a check. But he paid me about a fourth of what he owed. He had promised I would receive fifty percent of everything I billed. When he saw the numbers I was putting on the books, he told me I must have misunderstood the arrangement and it would be fifty percent of everything collected. "Don't worry about the money," he said. I was the new kid on the block and wasn't supposed to make waves. He had been practicing medicine for thirty years, but in three months I had made more money than he ever did. His secretary said he simply didn't have the money in his corporate account to pay me all we had contracted.

I continued vacation coverage for the other practices. I decided that after my commitment was fulfilled, I wanted to be on my own. I certainly didn't want to join these doctors. The patients were less than exciting and had too many foot problems. If I had wanted to do this type of work, I would have become a podiatrist. These offices were packed full of patients who had had bunion operations and their toes had become crooked again. People by the dozens came in to have their corns removed. I saw multiple sores on heels that were growing larger by the visit.

After three months, I had built a large enough practice from doctor referrals that I didn't need these practices. I hired our secretary from the residents' office at the university and she helped me get started. She was sick of the bureaucracy at the university and couldn't wait to leave.

But I hadn't noticed who was watching my expanding practice. My good buddy Dr. Cataract had an office only a few blocks from the hospital, and the nurses in the emergency room told me that he stopped by every morning to see what patients had been admitted the night before with orthopedic problems and to see which doctor they had been referred to. He scolded an emergency room doctor one morning for not following the call list.

These poor emergency room doctors were tired of waiting two to three hours for an orthopedist like Dr. Cataract to call them back or show up. So they started doing what made sense. They called someone who would come in to take care of the problem immediately. Let's face it, the people in the emergency room had a logistics problem. They had patients that needed to be admitted and the quickest way was to call a doctor who would respond. They knew that if they called me and a patient needed admission, they would have another bed available within half an hour. But I had done something wrong. I had gotten busy—the ultimate sin for a newcomer in Dr. Cataract's community.

I was told by one emergency room doctor that Dr. Cataract was looking for trouble and the emergency room doctors were going to back off calling me for a while. I was furious. What had I done? I had come into the hospital day and night, had taken good care of the patients, and this was the thanks I got?

Then the axe fell when I ran into Dr. Cataract in the parking lot. He stopped me to say that it was his duty as the orthopedic chief of the hospital to keep tabs on all new orthopedists in the community. He said it was time to review my charts because I was accumulating a lot of patients much more quickly than any young orthopedist had in the past. I asked him if there was a problem. He turned away without looking me in the eye, got into his car, and left.

The next day I ran into an emergency room nurse and she asked me what the notice on the emergency room bulletin board meant. I said I didn't know anything about it. We walked to the emergency room briskly as she mentioned something about my privileges being restricted until all of my charts had been reviewed by Dr. Cataract. I broke out in a cold sweat.

As I read the notice, my fists became clenched. He couldn't do that. I hadn't done anything wrong. I hadn't committed a crime. But I had. I had committed the ultimate sin. I had taken big bucks out of Dr. Cataract's pocket. Who was going to pay for his new cars every year?

I called him on the phone but he wouldn't talk to me. He was "with a patient." I called the chief of staff, who told me that Dr. Cataract had informed him that I might have some problems. "Dr. Cataract thinks we need to slow you down a little bit," he said. I was incensed. How could I possibly have my privileges restricted and a notice put up on the bulletin board about me without even being notified and allowed to respond to this charge? The chief of staff agreed that this was the incorrect protocol and that he would talk to Dr. Cataract. Wasn't I entitled to my day in court?

The next few months would be the worst of my life. I was a condemned man. Dr. Cataract had hung a WANTED sign on me. Rumors jetted around town that I was being reviewed like a parolee.

I had all I could do not to strangle Dr. Cataract. He began writing letters on hospital stationery asking me questions like, "On August 4, you performed hip surgery on Mrs. Demetre. In your operative report, you stated that you incised the muscle but you didn't say it was closed at the end of surgery. Can you explain this to the committee?" Committee? Now Dr. Cataract had formed a posse to lynch me, to get me out of town.

I explained in a letter that it was customary to close all muscles in a wound after fixing the hip but he scolded me for not mentioning it in my operative report. That was strange because I had reviewed several of Dr. Cataract's operative reports while at Aggie University and most of his reports were barely six sentences long. Sometimes it was even difficult to tell which operation Dr. Cataract had done because his reports were so brief.

The badgering continued for the next several weeks. I continued to receive letters from Dr. Cataract about things I had done or not done in the past few months. No matter what I said, it was wrong and I would be reprimanded. They wanted me out at any cost. They were willing to sacrifice their integrity and lie about the standard of care in the orthopedic surgery community in order to get rid of the guy who was draining money out of their pension plans.

Another patient they reviewed was a young man who had dismounted inappropriately from his motorcycle and fractured his thigh bone. Rather than making him hang in traction for six weeks and have his bone heal crooked, which was the standard of care for this medical community, I rodded his femur and he was up and walking in two days. He left the hospital within six days and the fracture healed in six weeks. But since the average age of the orthopedic staff was about sixty and no one had ever been trained to rod thigh bones, I was reprimanded and scolded for being so surgically aggressive. "We noticed your patient with the broken femur had postoperative films that showed a fracture that was not there in the preoperative x-rays. Can you explain this?" Dr. Cataract wrote.

I initially wrote that if he would have bothered to look, he would have noticed two fractures. But my better judgment took over and I explained it was common to break off a tiny chip of bone at the fracture site as the rod was passing through the bone. I even persuaded my old chief, who was a noted trauma expert in the country, to write a letter of support. But the committee disregarded his letter and reemphasized that rodding a femur was not the state of the art in Dr. Cataract's community. I had fractured the leg worse than it was—even though the patient got an excellent result. They said I should have hung the little fellow in traction and let him rot for six weeks, like all of their patients. You know, run the bill up to about $30,000 and give the patient a few bed sores by which to remember the experience.

I eventually got a letter from this highly ethical mob saying they would like to meet with me to discuss these cases. Dr. Airhead told me it would help my cause at the hearing if I said, "Yes, sir" and "No, sir" to everything that was asked of me. I said, "Yes, sir." "Don't be defensive," he said. But why not? They only wanted to destroy my life and kick me out of town.

We all met the next day. They sat me down at a long table and I looked around to notice all eyes peering at me. They explained that a review of my cases showed I was too aggressive surgically. It didn't make any difference that I achieved excellent results or that my patients were happy. I was merely too good for their mediocre medical community and I'd better stop it immediately. None of my answers to their inquiries were adequate and they all agreed that they were ashamed of my aggressive performance. I was told to clean up my act.

I had had it. What would I accomplish by remaining in this community? I hadn't slept for three months because of this torture. I wasn't eating. I was a good orthopedist but I was miserable, and I didn't want to be surrounded by these mental derelicts anymore.

My referring doctors told me to hang in there and this lynching mob would retreat. I was told that this same group had tried to do this to every young orthopedist who came to town. I had brought it to a head because it was a good time to criticize someone after the hospital administration had been nationally embarrassed by the previously mentioned anesthesiology scandal. So it was my hand they decided to slap even though I was a competent orthopedic surgeon who got good results.

There was something else that added to my popularity during this war. I frequently attended high school football games on Friday and Saturday nights. I did this to make a little extra money and to meet different coaches and trainers in the community so they might send me business. And it worked. I frequently got cases from the games and many of the schools started using me as their team physician.

I also met two people during this football season who would add to the medical community's hatred of me. One was a local sports reporter for a big newspaper. We struck up a conversation at one of the local high school football games. He decided he wanted to do an article on a sports doctor. He wrote an article about me, emphasizing all of my previous professional football affiliations. There was a huge picture of me. I noticed all of my competitors in town barely spoke to me for weeks after its publication. Dr. Round rudely approached me to say, "Gee, nice piece of advertisement in the local paper, Doctor."

The other bit of sin I committed for a newcomer was that I met a local television sportscaster at a playoff high school football game. He had seen the article about me in the paper and was favorably impressed. He further explained that he was new in town and the station where he worked was having some trouble with ratings. Back East he had just completed a short series on sports injuries, and he wondered if I would be interested in doing such a "mini series" with him. I was open for business. And I hadn't seen the posse gathering for several weeks. So we got together and produced a series on running injuries called "Running for the Health of It."

We shot scenes in my office and in various locations in town. We did a segment about appropriate shoe wear in a store selling running shoes. He interviewed some of my patients with running injuries. We even filmed a segment in surgery as we operated on the news director at his station. The entire series was well done and we approached air time with great anticipation. I was looking for business and he was looking for ratings. We weren't disappointed. The station's ratings rose significantly and it did wonders for his popularity with the station. At the same time my referrals were also increasing. This was done at a very opportune time in the exercise world, when running was reaching its peak with young and old alike. We interviewed an older gentleman with shin splints and did another segment on children's orthopedics. Of course runners aren't great surgical cases and they don't fall and break lots of bones, but business is business. And that was what I needed. Or did I?

I went to grand rounds at the university and happened to sit next to Dr. Mac, who was still the chief of orthopedics at the local prepaid health plan. He asked me how it was going out in the community and told me he had heard how I was being harassed. He mentioned how his group now had about 300,000 members and how badly they needed a young orthopedist, especially one trained in arthroscopy. He added I could average doing about ten arthroscopies a week at the Free For All Clinic and he couldn't understand why I needed all this other political nonsense. I had gotten tired over the years of hearing Dr. Mac's sermons, but it dawned on me that he might be right for once.

I could go to the Free For All Clinic, do my thing, and put this whole nightmare behind me. I cringed at the thought of giving in to these vultures, but at what expense did I want to fight? No sleep. No time for my family. No happiness. I decided to quit and take his offer.

For several months I felt very torn and that I had really failed. Why didn't I stay and fight? I could have won. On the other hand, I felt relieved, like the world had just climbed off my shoulders. I no longer had to deal with Dr. Cataract. He was incompetent, dishonest, and poorly respected. But he beat me this round. He had too much power. I no longer had to worry about billing or collecting, just practicing orthopedic surgery. My secretary cried when I first told her the news. She had worked hard and supported me until the bitter end. She reminded me I had always been a fighter and not to stop now. But it was ruining my life. I had to eat crow this time.

I thought about suing the hospital. I even talked to a close friend of my parents who was an aggressive personal injury attorney, but my case didn't offer him a large enough settlement. And my other concern was that if I sued a doctor at this time in my career, when I still hadn't taken my Boards, I probably would be blackballed. That could be a serious problem for me in the future should I want to get back into the private practice world.

I already had one mark against me. Remember, Dr. Cataract had restricted my privileges in the emergency room, which meant I was officially reported to the local medical quality assurance board. This would remain on my record for five years. I was scared.

I had definitely made some money and a lot more would be coming in over the next several months from my accounts receivable. I had made in a few months what I would make in two years at the Free For All Clinic. But money wasn't everything. Remember that's what Dr. Round told me when he cheated me out of all that money.

I realized that for several months I would have to maintain a low profile and simply drown in my sorrow. I knew that everyone was talking about me and how I was kicked out of town. It hurt badly. But I felt with time it would pass. So I closed my office, took down my sign, sold my equipment, forwarded my mail to my home address, and headed off for the next venture in my life at the Free For All Clinic. I had lost this battle but not the war. All because I wanted to be a doctor.

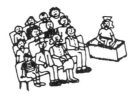

16. Free For All Clinic

MY FIRST DAY on the job at the Free For All Clinic was amusing. I needed to learn an entirely new system and there were dozens of new faces and places with which I would need to become familiar in a hurry. I first went to meet with Dr. Mac. He reassured me that I was really needed here and he would be keeping a close eye on my performance. Although he attempted to make me feel somewhat small, I knew this was just his style and he meant no harm.

He then introduced me to the rest of the orthopedists and their assistants. You can't imagine the variety of human beings here. This was a group of docs who didn't want to go out and make the grade in private practice. They preferred to just sit back and skate into retirement, doing the least amount of work possible for a paycheck. Most of the staff were elderly. I was clearly on a different mission. I was there to do a lot of cases, to become proficient in arthroscopy, and then to leave.

The first orthopedist I met was Dr. Nick. I could barely see his face through the thick cloud of smoke from his cigarette. He was direct and let me know that he was old and tired and every good case he found in clinic, he would gladly give me. In addition, he offered to pay me to do any of his night call. This seemed generous to me. I left coughing on my way to the next introduction.

Dr. Mumbles was a fat black doctor who jumbled all of his words together in one sentence. He let me know that he had a significant amount of experience in sports medicine and knee surgery. He told me he was the in-house expert in the field and had been for a long time. He also was willing to rid himself of any call that might interest me.

Between introductions I learned that all doctors had to keep time sheets for their hours, like clerks in a grocery store. Even more complicated, we had to specify whether the hours were spent in surgery, clinic, or meetings. This would turn out to be a royal pain in the ass. We had to do it every day and couldn't just fill out the whole thing at the end of the month. I couldn't remember to do this so I just put down whatever I thought looked good. Screw 'em.

Other notables I met included Dr. Show, a large female who combed her hair straight back. She raised large dogs as a hobby. She was very pleasant but I was told that she was late to everything—meetings, surgery, and clinic. It was funny to chat with her. Every ten minutes she would whip out a breath freshener from her white coat and spray it in her mouth. But this was necessary because she smoked. I was dying to ask her if it would be too much trouble to stop by the offices of Drs. Nick and Mumbles every half hour and spray their mouths too. But I thought that might be too presumptuous on my first day.

Dr. Deal was a retired military man who primarily practiced hand surgery. He was an excellent orthopedist and a good teacher, making complicated hand problems understandable. He often helped me reason out difficult cases. Since he had definite aspirations to being the next department chief, he made sure he was on all the right hospital committees.

I was afraid of Dr. Deal because he was extremely moody and often lost his temper, sometimes with other doctors and sometimes with his patients. He had one great line which I have never forgotten: "If you cut, you cry." He explained that sooner or later, no matter how good a surgeon you might be, you'll have complications, a bad result, a stiff knee, a fracture that doesn't heal. You'll be sued and involved in all kinds of litigation.

After I met the rest of the team, I was led to the little cubbyhole they called my office. It was a six-by-eight-foot cell, but it did have a view of the parking lot. Next I met my assistant, Jesus. He was a Mexican gentleman, about forty years old. I was told that he wasn't too smart but tried very hard. He told me he was looking forward to being with a new doctor in the department and would do anything he could to help me. He seemed friendly and energetic and he didn't smoke.

I met the seventy-year-old registered nurse who answered telephone calls from patients. She was called the advice nurse. The patients hated her because she never let them talk to the doctor and she always had an answer for everything, no matter what. She could have stopped a DC-10 on takeoff with her looks. She wore a nurse's cap, stood about four feet tall, and her teeth stuck out past her nose.

My first day she stopped by my office to review the day's schedule. She reminded me, "Don't take too long with any one patient or you'll get behind." At the Free For All Clinic we were assigned a patient every fifteen minutes, whatever the problem. It worked out because for a follow-up visit only about five minutes were needed, unless the patient needed an x-ray, which took an eternity.

My final introduction was to the physician in charge of the whole operation, Dr. Done. He was tall, bald, and smoked a pipe. He was a fast talker who assured me that with my potential, I could quickly climb the ladder of success at the Free For All Clinic.

During the first day I had an opportunity to sit down with the charge nurse of the clinic, Greta. She was a giant of a woman. She was big, tall, and ugly, perfect for the job. She told me what she expected from my slot in the clinic and she conveyed that she kept close tabs on the productivity of each doctor. I felt like I was back in grade school. I knew right away that she and I would not become bosom buddies.

Finally, I met Becky, who scheduled the surgeries. She told me, "Tuesday morning and Friday afternoon are your days for surgery and Thursday afternoon you assist." It didn't sound like a lot of time if I was expected to do most of the arthroscopy, but I would see. She said if I needed more operating time I might be able to take Dr. Nick's slot. "In those cases, you take his operating time and he goes down to clinic and sees your patients," she explained. But wait a minute. My patients won't want to see him. They'll want to see me. Becky explained it wasn't a problem, because Free For All Clinic patients rarely saw the same doctor when they came in, like it or not.

I went down to the laundry room where I was told to pick up my white coats, even though I didn't like wearing them. It scared the kids. I thought doctors who wore white coats were stuffy and trying to play a role. We didn't get dirty seeing patients. It was stupid. My patients had always been more relaxed because I didn't wear a white coat. But I got lucky. They spelled my name wrong so I pitched them all.

I also stopped by the mail room and introduced myself. Then I ran up to the orthopedic ward to meet the people who took care of the in-house patients. The head nurse was a very talkative lady who was excited that a younger doctor was here. She told me how she had to make rounds with the older docs because they couldn't remember their patients. On her days off some of the patients wouldn't be seen for two days. I was wondering what happened when she went on vacation.

It was lunchtime and I was told to be back by 1:00 p.m. It happened that my first day was also a noon staff meeting for all the doctors and I was invited to attend. I went and everyone was very gracious about introducing me to the other physicians. I was starting to feel like one of the clan. I grabbed a tray and got into the buffet line. The food looked and smelled like dog food. But I didn't want to give any negative feedback so I went heavy on the milk and salad.

The topic of the day was group business. I listened as Dr. Done told the partners that because they had cut down on the number of lab tests they ordered and because the surgeons had operated less this year, the bonuses for all would be higher than anticipated. I was flabbergasted. Did I hear this correctly? The money that these folks made was dependent on whether or not they did or did not order tests or do surgery? Did that mean that maybe, just maybe, surgeries that were indicated on some were not performed because the doctors knew their bonuses would be bigger? I must have misinterpreted what I heard. I would find out more later.

Jesus was waiting for me at my office and seemed excited about us working together. He couldn't wait to put the patients in the rooms and he was willing to learn things my way. I was eager to let him participate if he paid attention and showed an interest. I was told that all the young doctors in the past seven years had come and gone within a year. I explained to Jesus that I wanted him to work with me rather than for me. I said that I liked to move very fast and that I didn't have a lot of patience. If he could help me with all the paperwork and get people in and out of the rooms quickly, we would generally be done before quitting time. He seemed organized and anxious to get started.

Promptly at 1:00 p.m. we started to see patients. Most of them had bread-and-butter orthopedic problems and, as I had expected, there were several people with negative tales of past treatment at the clinic. I hoped to change all that over time. By the end of the day, I had filled all of my surgery slots for two weeks—two locked knees, one recurrent shoulder dislocation, and a lady with severe degenerative arthritis of the knee. If you liked to operate, this was the place.

My first week was a real eye-opener. There was so much orthopedic pathology in this place I couldn't believe it. All kinds of cases: total joint replacement, knee arthroscopy, trauma, you name it. I began to think that all residents just out of training should be obligated to spend time in a place like this for at least two years to get some experience doing good cases without having to beg for referrals from other doctors. The salary was decent and you could perfect the skills you had learned in training.

The first Friday morning was the weekly x-ray conference when the entire department presented the patients on the orthopedic ward. It was amusing to see what really turned on some of the staff members. Dr. Stripes stood up and showed an x-ray of a routine hip fracture. This was everyday orthopedics to most but he looked and sounded like he had just found a cure for cancer. Then it suddenly dawned on me that things moved a little slower here and that the docs were behind the current trends. I presented a lady who had a hip replacement and Dr. Mac immediately asked me what type of prosthesis I had used as it didn't look like one out of the surgery set. I explained that this prosthesis was the type I had used in my residency and it was the state of the art in orthopedics today. The equipment man was happy to bring by the entire set and the Free For All Clinic would just be charged for the prosthesis, not the equipment rental.

Dr. Mac was angry. He explained that the reason the department used the current set was that the company gave the hospital a significantly reduced price if the doctors agreed to use this prosthesis exclusively. He was obviously afraid that if it were found that I was using another type, the Free For All Clinic would lose their deal. He said, "This could cost the partnership down the road." Was I hearing the same theme I heard at conference? Did he want me to use equipment I was uncomfortable or unfamiliar with? He said we would talk about it later. I sat down and felt I had been severely scolded in front of my peers on my first presentation. Was this a sample of what was to come? At least Dr. Nick mentioned that the prosthesis looked like it was in excellent position.

Later that afternoon Dr. Mac stopped by as I was writing in a chart. "Let's talk a few minutes, Buck," he said as we went into my office and closed the door. "Buck, listen, I want you to understand clearly what I was trying to tell you this morning. If everyone in the department were using a different type of equipment, we couldn't save any money and it would cost the partnership a mint. After all, in orthopedics, we use more equipment than any other surgical specialty, so we have to cut costs somewhere." Here we go again. I explained to him that we had tried all of the different prostheses at the university and it was felt by all the professors that on the total joint service the one I had used was far superior to any other. I really had to use the one I thought best for my patient.

He could see I would not concede, so he agreed to speak with the personnel in the surgery supply room. But he warned me, if my equipment couldn't be purchased at the present rate, I might not be able to do total joints in the future at the Free For All Clinic. It didn't make any difference that I was the most recently trained or that I had just spent six months on the total joint service. Not only that, most of the doctors on staff were so old that they weren't trained to do total joints. And these surgeries were so long and stressful that the docs couldn't complete an entire case without getting chest pains or pooling of blood in their leg veins.

I wanted to explore another problem with Dr. Mac. "Correct me if I'm wrong, but I thought the main reason I was brought here was to do arthroscopy. Yesterday I went and reviewed the equipment here and you are in desperate need of at least $20,000 worth of tools." As expected, I was told that it would be nice if I could make do with what the hospital already had. "Besides, for the next two years there is no more money in the budget for orthopedic equipment," he explained with a smile.

I decided I had made enough waves my first week. But there was absolutely no way that I would agree to use inferior instruments on patients for whose outcome I was ultimately responsible. After all, surgery was stressful enough even if you had the right tools under the right circumstances.

I received a call to stop by the bookkeepers' office to sign some employment papers. She was located in Dr. Done's suite so I thought I'd watch my step and make sure I didn't run into him. The book-keeper was a pleasant lady. We discussed my salary and deductions at length and when we were finished, she asked a question I had been asked at least ten times in the past week: "What is a nice young doctor doing in a place like this when you could be making so much more money in private practice?"

I walked out the door only to run into Dr. Done who was heading out with his briefcase. "How are things going, Buck?" he asked. I told him that things were great and I was honored to be part of the Free For All Clinic. I felt like I was back in my medical school interviews.

The next several months determined my longevity at the clinic. Most of the patients were healthy, and I had no complaints. I saw lots of interesting orthopedic problems and got plenty of surgical experience. I became so inundated with cases that I was having to tell patients it would be three to four months before I could replace their hips or remove the ganglion from their wrists. I couldn't get any more operating time and I really didn't understand why until I investigated the problem thoroughly.

I learned that each person in the department had the same amount of operating time but there were only a few of us doing all the surgery. It seemed that the older, slower doctors would book in two very small cases for a four hour block and tell the scheduling clerk that that was the most they could handle in one day. We younger guys did three to four big cases in the same time slot. I spoke to the surgery supervisor who had taken a liking to me. She told me what I didn't want to hear.

It seemed that these doctors would show up at about 2:00 p.m. for a 1:00 p.m. case, and then when they were finished they would go into the lounge area for a few cigarettes and then do the last case and finish about 4:00 p.m. The block was scheduled until 5:00 p.m. They would then promptly leave and no one would know the difference. So my patients were waiting three to four months for surgery because these guys didn't want to work or release this time to the rest of us. They went up to surgery to relax and to avoid clinic. Clinic required them to see twenty patients and that was too stressful. I was catching on.

Yes, clinic was stressful. Patients whom I saw at 1:30 p.m. and sent to x-ray would not return until 3:30 or 4:00 p.m. Jesus would run down there frequently, only to find a huge line. You would think that orthopedics would have their own x-ray unit, but not at the Free For All Clinic.

I decided I would check it out on my own, starting at registration. I walked through the x-ray waiting room that was filled to the brim with at least one hundred people, and I strolled up to the man at the desk. I started to introduce myself when he told me very bluntly to wait my turn.

A frightened young lady handed the receptionist a slip of paper and said, "My doctor sent me here for a mammogram because I have a lump in my breast." He tore off one of the sheets, gave her back her slip, and said, "It will be a few minutes, so please have a seat behind the lady in the red dress who is having a hysterectomy in the morning." I couldn't believe this insensitive and impersonal situation. Everyone around the desk felt equally awkward.

This would soon be topped. As my turn approached, a young x-ray technician appeared, grabbed the microphone, and announced, "Everyone here waiting to have a barium enema, please follow me through the blue door."

I was outraged. Was nothing sacred anymore? Why didn't we have each person in the waiting room come up to the microphone one at a time and announce his ailment?

The obnoxious receptionist left for a break and a gorgeous young lady stepped up to the desk and asked if she could help me. She had long black hair with a beautiful face and long, skinny legs. I told her who I was and asked if someone would show me around the department. She handed some slips to her assistant and asked me to come around through the door. "For a new doctor, you seem very busy already," she remarked. She showed me the rather unimpressive x-ray facilities and I told her about the incredible wait my patients were experiencing. She told me that two hours for routine films was normal and the patients expected this. She suggested that I send all of my patients needing an x-ray early because the first ones in were usually the first ones out.

I wasn't happy about the whole setup, but her idea seemed to make sense and I told her I would have Jesus start this procedure immediately. She added, "You seem like a real nice guy, so we'll see to it that your patients get through here just a little bit faster." I told her how much I appreciated her help. As I was getting ready to leave, she asked me if I would look at her ankle, which she had sprained playing soccer. I told her it would be best to tape the ankle and I offered to do so when she got off work. She smiled and said she would be there immediately after five. X-ray was like a rat maze and I barely found my way back to the orthopedic department.

My next thrill came when I paid a visit to the cast room later in the day. I was told by Jesus that the patients waited there for at least an hour to be seen. This backup was due to patients dropping by the clinic without an appointment because their casts were broken. Scores of emergency room patients were sent over for a cast or a splint. But I knew it only took about ten minutes to put one on and about thirty seconds to cut one off. Something was wrong. I went off to investigate.

At least the cast room was located in the orthopedic department. This would suggest that someone had a few brain cells working when this whole operation was originally planned. There were ten chairs outside the cast room and these were occupied. There were four stalls for casting but only three were being used by cast technicians. The other was left open for physicians who wanted to come over and do their own work.

As a patient hobbled out of a stall with her crutches, I asked the tech why there were so many people waiting. He responded, "Well, Dr. Mays, we have to do all of the casts from our own twelve doctors, plus all of the casts sent over from the emergency room, plus casts for patients who get theirs wet or broken."

I asked, "What percentage of your work is for patients returning with broken casts?" I was told about thirty percent. Then I learned that the cast material being used was plaster of paris. Clearly, the new generation of orthopedics dictated the use of fiberglass. It was stronger, lighter, waterproof—and more expensive.

When I inquired about this policy, I was told fiberglass was too costly and the administration would not hear of such a drastic change. That made no sense at all. Fiberglass casts were more expensive, yes, but they lasted much longer than plaster because they were harder and waterproof. So when the patients got them wet, they didn't need constant changing like diapers. In other words, if you put the increased cost of the casting material up against the excessive number of cast changes required for broken or wet plaster casts, it would be cost-effective to use fiberglass. Right?

I asked two of the cast technicians about my philosophy and they told me not to waste my breath. They had tried approaching the powers that be and this idea had fallen on deaf ears. The technicians agreed that fiberglass was less messy and would virtually eliminate the two-hour cleanup required by housekeeping each night.

I wondered why so many people tolerated such medical care. One reason was obvious, most people just didn't know any better. The Free For All Health Plan was given free to workers of the state and city. The private plans took additional monies out of employees' paychecks. But even so, wouldn't it be better to pay a few more bucks and be able to choose your own doctor, not have to sit in waiting rooms filled with thirty people, and not have to wait in x-ray for two hours for a sixty-second chest x-ray? Why would people want to wait three months for an elective surgery when a private surgeon could perform the same procedure at a newly built hospital the same week of your request?

I had so many patients waiting in x-ray that I had nothing to do, so I decided to slip over to the candy machine by the pharmacy for a chocolate fix. What was going on? They must be giving away free drugs. I recognized one of my patients sitting in the back of the large pharmacy waiting room. "Oh, hi, Dr. Mays," she groaned. "I turned in my prescription and I'm waiting for my number to be called." She showed me her red sixty-four. I looked over and saw they were on number forty-three. It then occurred to me that I had seen this lady in clinic before lunch, approximately three hours ago. I shook my head, patted her on the back, and wandered away in disbelief.

Her six-year-old son cried for her to take him home. I went back and asked her if it would be all right if I took him over to the candy machine with me. She thanked me profusely. I bought him a Milky Way. He would have time to fly there and back before his mother would be ready to leave.

The Free For All Clinic was not stupid when they recruited me. I was naive and I didn't understand the system. I worked myself into a rut. I was so busy that I worked from 7:00 a.m. to 8:00 p.m. when I wasn't on call. Since I was trying to earn extra money, I was on call about twice a week and didn't get home those nights until about midnight. These late nights were often followed by three or four elective surgery cases the next morning at 7:30.

One night I was waiting in the emergency room for a patient to return from x-ray. A nurse who had taken a liking to me for setting her son's wrist fracture started to rub my neck muscles while I wrote orders at the nurses' station. As I moaned my approval, she said, "You really don't understand the system, do you?" I turned around and looked at her with my bloodshot eyes and asked her what she meant. She continued, "All you young aggressive guys come to the Free For All Clinic and get screwed. You have lots of energy so you work at the lowest possible salaries while the partners draw the big bucks. They know they get paid the same whether they work hard or not. So they send you all the good cases and you think they're doing you a favor. You're so busy doing all these cases and taking so much call that you burn out at a young age without realizing what you're doing to yourself physically and emotionally."

She was right. I was frustrated, tired, and making very little money. Just so I could be busy. Just so I could do the most cases in the department. And all the partners were sitting back in their big easy chairs laughing.

As I walked back to my office I passed Dr. Mumbles's office and glanced at his schedule for tomorrow morning. He had a total of six patients that started at 9:30 a.m. and he was finished at 11:15 a.m. I strolled back to my counter and noticed I had two surgical cases from 7:30 a.m. until 9:30 a.m. and then fifteen patients from 9:30 a.m. until noon.

I stormed over to look at Dr. Nick's schedule for tomorrow. He was in a deposition all day. Depositions started at 10:00 a.m. and rarely went beyond noon. Why couldn't he see patients from 9:00 a.m. to 10:00 a.m.? What the hell was he going to be doing all afternoon?

I glanced at my watch and noticed it was 11:00 p.m. I quickly grabbed the messages on my desk and headed for the parking lot. As I drove home, I reviewed my messages. The head of medical records had called and said I had twenty delinquent charts to sign. Another one said that my patient Mrs. Avery had called to say she was out-raged that it would take six weeks to get her son on the operating schedule to remove the loose bodies floating around in his elbow.

The next message was from Mrs. Gomez, asking for my recom-mendation to a physical therapist outside the Free For All Clinic. She had tried to schedule an appointment for her low back pain and was told there were no openings for eight weeks. She could barely walk. She wanted a note saying she needed outside therapy so she could go to the administration at the Free For All Clinic and try to be reim-bursed. Good luck. And last, but not least, a familiar tune, Mrs. Casandra had called to say her little boy had gotten his plaster arm cast wet in the sprinklers and wondered if she could bring him in tomorrow for a new cast. What about fiberglass?

At this point I knew it was over. The die was cast. There was no way I could work much longer in this environment. Almost all of the patients were angry. Rightfully so. The quality of care was deter-mined by politics and money rather than by compassion and good medical judgment. I decided to take no more extra call at night for any of the partners and, effective immediately, I would accept no more patient referrals from anyone else in the department. I felt bad because this would severely compromise the quality of care given the patients, but I couldn't take this grueling schedule anymore. I was becoming a nervous wreck.

The next morning, I received a phone call from Dr. Done's office. He wanted to see me as soon as possible. Was I in trouble again? Had I offended someone? I called his office and was told to stop by that morning between patients. I did about 10:00 a.m., during a lull in the schedule waiting for my 8:30 a.m. patients to return from x-ray. I sat in his waiting room wondering what I had done wrong. I had been a little short at times with some of the incompetent staff and had possibly shared my disgust with the Free For All Clinic once too often with the patients. But I had never realized I was that bad.

Then he blasted through the door. "Come in, Doctor," he smiled. "Buck, I just thought it was time for us to have a chat. I've been keeping close tabs on you the last several months, especially in regard to patient satisfaction and the surgery schedule. It's clear to me that you are definitely the major producer in the orthopedic department and the patients seem to love you. I've decided to bypass all the usual committees and bureaucratic nonsense and give you a $25 a month bonus, effective immediately," he stated.

I was stunned. A $25 bonus, $300 a year? That was about one-sixth of what a private orthopedist earned for one arthroscopy that took fifteen minutes to perform. It was the price of a cheap pasta dinner for two. I wanted to tell him to stick it up his annoying humidifier that was blasting in the background. But I decided to use the occasion to my benefit.

"Thank you very much for this nice vote of confidence, Dr. Done. I have really enjoyed working at your hospital. But I wonder if I could put the money toward some new arthroscopic equipment that is badly needed in surgery. The equipment here is very outdated and has affected the quality of my arthroscopic procedures." He leaped out of his chair. "Why didn't you come to me with this problem before? I thought the whole reason we recruited you to this hospital centered on your expertise in arthroscopy?" he yelled. I explained that I had voiced my concerns to Dr. Mac but was told that since I was the only one doing arthroscopy, it was low priority in the departmental budget. Furthermore, it was no secret that Dr. Mac was not trained to use the arthroscope and he considered this procedure experimental.

Dr. Done's face was red as he groaned angrily and sat back in his chair. "How much do you need?" he asked. I told him it would take about $20,000 and he said that he would take it out of administrative funds. He told me to go ahead and order it immediately, and he thanked me for my dedication and hard work. I was told to come to him right away the next time I encountered this sort of difficulty or any other problem that needed his help.

I returned to the department feeling much better about my situation. But as I thought about it, what had changed really? As soon as I got the new toys I wanted, I would probably schedule more cases and work even harder. But I had been given a vote of confidence. Dr. Done liked me and the patients liked me too. Over the lunch hour I found all of the tools I wanted in catalogs and began calling the manufacturers myself. It was really fun shopping with someone else's money.

I hustled the patients in and out of clinic and then ran home to tell my wife how well I was liked at the Free For All Clinic. The bonus was a joke, and the equipment was a mere token so I would keep producing, but the positive feedback made me feel needed and important. After a wonderful dinner, I settled into bed with my wife. I wasn't on call. What a pleasant change.

The phone rang at 2:00 a.m. I was sleeping so soundly that I grabbed for the receiver, knocking it on the floor. It was the hospital operator. "Dr. Mays, this is operator number three at the Free For All Clinic and I have an emergency call for you from surgery. Please hold." What the hell is she talking about? I'm not on call.

"Hello, Dr. Mays. This is Sheila from surgery. Sorry to bother you so late, but Dr. Adopt asked me to call you. He's scrubbed and in surgery, repairing a forearm from a plate glass window accident. But he's sick to his stomach and has been throwing up. He can't finish the case. There's a tourniquet around the patient's arm. He was wondering if you could come in to relieve him?"

At first I thought it was a dream. It couldn't be true. This was the kind of heroics you see on television. But I realized it was real. My wife awakened as I began stumbling around for some pants. I told her to go back to sleep and I would explain later. Much later.

I ran three red lights and got to the hospital in eight minutes. I quickly changed into my surgical scrubs and rushed into the operating room. Dr. Adopt turned to me. I could see his mask was soiled and the air smelled of vomit. I quickly glanced at the patient's forearm, which was filleted open on the table like a war wound. "Thanks so much for coming in, Buck," he said. "I must have the flu or something, and I didn't know who else to call who lived as close as you. I'm sorry for the inconvenience," he apologized.

He explained that this patient was drunk at a party and had fallen through a plate glass window. Seven tendons and two nerves were cut. Although he had identified and tagged all of them, none had been sewn up, and the tourniquet had already been on for one hour. I went out to quickly scrub my hands and told Dr. Adopt to go home and get some sleep.

I spent the next few minutes identifying his landmarks and then proceeded to sew the tendons and nerves back together. After twenty-five minutes I let the tourniquet down and amazingly there was very little bleeding, except for one artery that started shooting blood. I quickly clamped and tied it. I spent the next half hour doing a plastic closure so this rather attractive young lady wouldn't have to stare at an ugly scar the rest of her life. The problems she would face with hand function over the next several years would be enough of a reminder.

After I placed a large bandage and splint on her arm and wrote the orders, I sat back at the dictaphone machine to try and digest what had happened to me over the past few hours. The circulating nurse invited me into the nurses' lounge for a cup of coffee.

It was now 4:30 in the morning. She patted me on the back and said, "In the nineteen years I've been in the operating room, I've never seen anything like that. I was standing in the corner charting notes when I heard something that sounded like a loud dog bark. The vomiting spell hit Dr. Adopt so quickly that he would have thrown up into the wound had his mask not been on. Then Dr. Adopt fell to the ground. I tell you, Dr. Mays, I thought he was having a heart attack. The anesthesiologist helped me turn him on his back. He continued to throw up in his mask."

I joked, "It was lucky that the patient was asleep rather than under an arm block or she might have jumped up off the table and run away from this circus." Apparently Dr. Adopt had felt much better after throwing up the first time, so he scrubbed again, regowned, gloved, went back in, and threw up again.

Over the next few days word spread around the hospital that I was a hero. I had come out of the night to save a surgeon in distress. It would have all been worth it had Dr. Done offered me another $25 a month in bonuses.

I was starting to put my job at the Free For All Clinic in perspective. Yes, I had received some great strokes over the past few days but I couldn't help thinking what would happen to my relationship with Dr. Mac when he found out I had sidestepped him to get my arthroscopic equipment. He would feel powerless over me and that would be the end of our working relationship.

An increasing number of associates in the hospital felt that Dr. Mays should be chief. I heard it frequently. Dr. Mac hated being overshadowed by anyone, let alone a lowly newcomer like me. He frequently reminded me that I was a relatively inexperienced orthopedic surgeon, even with my arthroscopic skills. He insisted that I didn't need the latest and fanciest equipment to practice my skills.

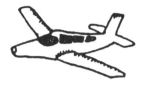

17. The Boards

HOW MANY hoops must one jump through? How much schooling must one endure before making it? Well, one day a bunch of old has-beens with nothing better to do gathered around a big table to establish the American Board of Bone Surgeons. Membership could only be obtained by passing an oral and written examination.

Let's face it. It would seem far too practical to fire a resident in an orthopedic training program who was failing to make the grade. Logic would dictate that if a resident were incompetent, dangerous, unreliable, or dishonest, the program chief could simply dismiss him. That was not the way it was.

It was generally accepted politically and academically that if a residency didn't graduate the same number of residents with which it started, there was something wrong with the program. It was inferior or it didn't have enough work to satisfy all the residents. Maybe the material at the hospital wasn't diversified enough to keep young doctors interested. These high and mighty academicians would never stoop so low as to say they had made a mistake or had misjudged an applicant.

Just try to find a program chief who tells you a facility doesn't have adequate staff to teach the residents or that the material in the program isn't well rounded enough to train the physicians. You won't. They don't exist. In academics the professors are perfect.

Well, at the end of your training you had to take the Board Exam to entitle you to be Board Certified in Orthopedic Surgery. Who cared, you ask? Nobody really. But it made the academicians happy that they had a Board and it made the profession look more legitimate. So you got to spend the last year of your residency being paranoid about this asinine test. In addition to all the stress of your senior year, like running a service, keeping the junior residents in line, and dealing with all the professors, you had to begin studying for the Boards.

There were two parts to the Boards. One was oral and one was written. As you can imagine, there was no shortage of advice from the professors and community doctors on how to study.

Some suggested going to a refresher course for three or four days. But really these were a quick fix. They were usually held in nice places like Hawaii, Palm Springs, or Florida, so the faculty could take a week off and fly first class. Each professor gave only a few lectures in order to justify his presence at the enrollees' expense. The courses generally cost around $1,000, which residents could hardly afford.

Others said, "Just read the orthopedic journals for the past five years and you'll know all you need to know for the exam." Still others said, "Just read your orthopedic textbooks and you'll be well prepared." No problem. These were only two huge volumes of material.

What did it mean to actually take the Boards and pass? What if you didn't pass? It was generally accepted by the medical community that you had reached the pinnacle of knowledge in your specialty if you passed the Boards. You could practice orthopedic surgery without the Boards, but you looked much better if you had made the grade.

Attorneys always asked you in depositions if you had your Boards. You certainly wouldn't be a very good witness if you had failed the Boards. Can you imagine spending eighty to one hundred hours a week for four to five years as a resident and this meaning absolutely nothing if you didn't pass a four-hour written test and two hours of oral interrogation? Yes, this is what medicine is all about: curriculum vitae, diplomas, and certificates.

Did it mean you were not a good orthopedic surgeon if you failed the Boards? The corollary to this frightened me the most. Did it mean that everyone who had passed the Boards was a good orthopedic surgeon? In this day and age, if you graduated from an approved residency program in this country, you were reasonably good at your specialty, whether you passed the Boards or not. But if you took the Boards ten or more years ago, you passed automatically because everyone did. It was the buddy system. All you had to do was show up. And I'll tell you what. Many of these doctors are still practicing today. They are poorly trained technically and performing surgeries that are outdated.

So what happened? Well, it seemed that the country became inundated with too many orthopedic surgeons graduating from all these programs. Wouldn't it make more sense to reduce the number of residencies or make the existing programs smaller? Wrong.

All the Board members, in their infinite wisdom, figured out the best way to control the saturation problem. Instead of letting it affect their comfortable academic positions, they decided to fail fifty percent of the residents who took the exam. The world would be told that only Board Certified Orthopedic Surgeons knew what they were doing.

All you had to do to be eligible to take the Boards was to kiss enough asses so a few doctors could write letters saying you were a good boy. What if someone wrote a less than complimentary letter about you to the Board? Did the Board check it out? Hell no. They just deferred your application another year. So if someone wanted to keep you out of the Boards, he could. It has been done. But blackballing doesn't exist anymore. Neither does sunshine.

And finally, how much did it cost every time you wanted to go on this ride? It was $500 to apply, $400 in airfare, $200 for a hotel, and another $300 in expenses.

My last year at the Free For All Clinic was, in part, spent preparing for the Boards. It was both good and bad that the doctor in the office next to me, Dr. Cappucino, was preparing for them too. The good news about this was that we could study together and console one another on a daily basis. We were a couple of smart guys who should pass. No problem. The bad news was that if we both didn't study as much as the other guy, we felt uncomfortable.

I decided to be my usual undisciplined self and not to take any time off to study before the Boards. I hoped for the best. I committed myself to studying every night before the Boards when I wasn't on call, about four times a week. Dr. Cappucino, on the other hand, took off three months from work to study before the Boards. Three months. A quarter of a year! This did nothing but increase my paranoia. There was absolutely no way I could study as much as he could. He would ace this test and I would look like a fool.

We had a plan for the final three months. He stayed home or went to the medical school library to study. I was in the clinic seeing patients or operating. Twice a week we would get together at night and go over orthopedic pathology slides of cysts, tumors, bone, and cartilage. One night a week, we jumped in the car and drove two hundred miles to review slides with a professor of orthopedic pathology. He showed us sections of tissues so we could make a diagnosis under a microscope.

Makes sense, doesn't it? Well, not really, when you consider that you would be hard-pressed to find one orthopedic surgeon in private practice in the United States who looks under a microscope. That's what pathologists do. They go through four years of residency looking under microscopes to be good at this. A practicing orthopedist never, and I mean never, looks at a slide. We don't even know how to adjust a microscope to see the tissue. We break slides trying to focus the stupid thing. If patients or their families ever had to depend on orthopedic surgeons for a microscopic diagnosis, the morbidity and mortality in orthopedics would quadruple.

For three months we kept this rigorous schedule. There were no exceptions or we'd run the risk of missing a few pages on the chemical content of cartilage that would surely be on the test. If we failed by one point, it would be because we took our wives out to dinner or the kids to the movie.

Both of us signed up for a refresher course in Bayview. It was only another $500. The lectures were boring and a complete waste of time, but the handout materials were good and could be studied in place of the lectures. So my schedule for each day differed from Dr. Cappucino's. I went to the lecture first thing in the morning, grabbed the handouts, and went to the coffee shop a block away to study. He sat through all the lectures, slept, and then went home at night and studied the handouts. Look at all the hours he wasted. Whatever turns you on.

As The Day approached, I asked some doctors who had passed the Boards for advice. "During the orals, what do you say if you flat out don't know the answer? Do you try to bullshit the examiner? Do you admit you don't know?" My wife suggested crying, which seemed to work well for her on the state nursing Boards. Most everyone I asked agreed that if you don't know something, say you don't know.

On the written test, however, it was much more complicated. The Board designed the test to reward you for correct answers and penalize you for wrong ones. If you were not sure, it would be best to leave it blank. But if you didn't get a certain number of questions right, you failed. So what do you do if you're eighty percent sure of the answer? How about sixty percent sure? This was going to be fun.

Dr. Cappucino and I agreed we would meet at the airport so our respective wives could bid us farewell before we left for the gas chamber. We got there about an hour early to check in and made sure we had seats on the plane. After we assured each other we would pass, we pulled out our notes and, yes, began studying again. Don't miss one moment of free time. Right?

Then an announcement came over the loudspeaker telling us our flight was overbooked and any passenger willing to wait two more hours for another flight would receive $300 in airline credit. We looked at each other and began to think. Hey, the test wasn't until tomorrow so what did we care whether we got there early tonight or late tonight? But Dr. Cappucino worried that the later flight might be delayed or worse, be cancelled, and then all of this studying would be for naught. We'd have to take the Boards a year later and send in another $500. "Let's not be foolish. I say no," he pleaded as I stroked my chin.

I went over to the ticket counter and asked the agent if he was reasonably sure the next flight would fly. He said the plane was already here and at the gate. He pleaded with me to switch because there were no takers and a lot of angry customers. I immediately recognized a potential deal as only I would. "I'll tell you what," I said. "If you guarantee me a first-class ticket and the $300 in credit, I'll help you out." He gave me a rather funny look and then glanced at his computer. "It looks like we have one seat left in first class so you've got yourself a deal. I like a man with imagination," he laughed. So do I.

He gave me my seat assignment, a $300 travel voucher, and thanked me. I headed back to a rather hostile Dr. Cappucino, not telling him about first class. He was disappointed but admitted I had more guts than he did. We went about our studying and agreed to meet when I arrived for a late dinner.

When the call came for him to board the plane, we shook hands and off he went. But with all the confusion of overselling the flight and people getting on and off the plane, they took off one hour and fifteen minutes late. I boarded my flight thirty minutes after he took off. Upon arrival in Chicago, the home of the Boards, his plane had a twenty-minute wait to get into a gate. My plane went directly to the gate assignment and unloaded. The net result of all this chaos was that I grabbed my luggage and ran for the waiting bus, finding Dr. Cappucino on the same bus. We had a good laugh. He just couldn't figure out why his flight served teriyaki chicken and mine served sautéed prime rib with wine. I felt good, as though this adventure might be an omen.

Chicago is always an experience in the summer. It was 98 degrees outside with 95 percent humidity. But what the hell. We weren't there to vacation. We were there on a mission, to pass the test and get the hell out of Dodge, as quickly as possible. I knew after this gig was over, I would be in no mood for any airline bargains. We got to our hotel, checked in, and headed for our rooms to shower. We agreed to meet in thirty minutes for dinner. Later we toured the various places in the hotel where we would be tested, so we knew just where to go. Then it was off to our rooms to study, one last time. This was our last chance to saturate our brain cells with this ridiculous data that we would remember for a few hours. Just so we could pass the test.

We got up two hours before we had to report. Dr. Cappucino and I met for breakfast and I could tell, as nervous as I was, he was petrified. He was spilling his coffee all over the saucer as he stirred in some cream. He dropped his spoon on the floor. I tried to console the both of us by saying, "This is what it's all about. It's the bottom of the ninth with the bases loaded and two outs. Let's go up to the plate and crash it over the fence."

All the applicants crowded into several different rooms for the briefing on the Board protocol. Some of us were to take the written test and some the orals the first day. I drew the written exam. I was told where to report and I did. What a pathetic-looking group of people.

All the applicants looked pale and sick. There was not a smile to be found. We all realized that every one of us was the other's enemy. Some would fail and some would pass, so I silently wished the worst for everyone in sight.

We were told that we were not to discuss anything about the exam with another person. If we met for dinner, we were to talk about something else, but not about the test. They reminded us that there was no reason to discuss it with friends. It would only give them an advantage. That was the first thing that made any sense to me.

I was happy to start with the written exam. It was the part of the test which made me the most uncomfortable because I knew it was mostly a guessing game. On the other hand, I could present myself well on the orals, even if I didn't know the right answer. After we were formally excused, I hustled back to my room to gain still a few more important facts before taking the final plunge.

The mixture of people in the room was alarming. Many were twenty to thirty years older than I, causing me to wonder if they had taken the test and previously failed. Or was this just their first time? Or were they trained in a foreign program and graduated later than others? No matter. Here I was and there they were and I couldn't concern myself with their stories. The test was finally handed out and we were told not to start until a bell was rung. The test was to take four hours. If you finished before that time, you had to sit there and wait for the full four hours. If you had to go to the restroom, you had to check out with the lady at the door, who would hold your test until you returned. And, of course, you had to keep your eyes on your own work or else. The bell rang.

The test was not easy. I was unsure of about thirty percent of the questions and I was having a great deal of trouble deciding whether to put an answer down or leave it blank. When I realized I had answered just three out of the first twenty, I decided I'd better get with the program and start having a little confidence.

It was a typical multiple-choice exam. I was not impressed with my knowledge and felt strongly that I had studied the wrong material. I had been told by many to study the basic sciences, like anatomy and physiology. But a large portion of the exam was on total joint replacement and hand surgery. Why had I listened to those idiots? I hadn't trusted them before I asked their advice, so why did I trust them at all? Why did I assume that the things that were emphasized last year would be the same this year? I should have assumed the opposite.

After three and a half hours of torture and frustration, I was finished and looked over my answer sheet. I felt squeamish about my performance and I was worried sick. Did I guess too much? Should I go over all two hundred questions again quickly? Forget it. I wanted out of there. I got up to leave, but one of the guards gave me a dirty look and reminded me it wasn't time. So I sat down and waited for the gong to sound.

It finally did, and they collected the papers. The fellow sitting next to me was penciling in one final answer when the examiner yanked his answer sheet out from under him, causing him to stroke a long lead line across his answer sheet. She hissed, "I hope that line doesn't cause the computer to spit out your exam."

I sulked all the way back to the room as I began wondering when I should begin studying for the Boards next year. I was sure I had failed. As I opened the door to my room, the phone rang. It was Dr. Cappucino. He sounded depressed and we decided to meet soon to take a walk around town. Before leaving I lay on the bed for a few minutes staring at the ceiling and reflected on what I had just been through. It wasn't fun. It was worse than I had heard. Was there any chance in hell I had passed? Probably not. But at least the written part was over and that felt good. I headed out the door to meet Dr. Cappucino.

He looked sick. "You'll never believe what happened to me this morning on the orals," he yelled. "You know that Dr. Cell, the bird-brain orthopedic pathologist that writes all those horrible articles in the literature? I got that turkey for my pathology orals. I walked into his little booth and recognized his face immediately. I was intimidated."

Dr. Cell had told him to sit down without even looking at him. No "Good morning" or handshake. Then Dr. Cell described a young female patient with an unusual growth on her leg and said, "Let's look at the microscopic slides together. Look at the pink area on the edge of the slide and tell me what tissue that is." Dr. Cappucino had answered that it looked like cartilage. "Is that what cartilage looks like, Doctor?" Dr. Cell questioned.

Two of his four orals were like that. Dr. Cappucino was discouraged that he had not been well coached. The examiners weren't interested in how he presented himself or the material. They just wanted the right answer.

I felt very bad. First of all, I felt bad for Dr. Cappucino. He had obviously gotten off on the wrong foot and I was afraid that this would affect his performance on the written exam. But worse, I was getting scared. I, too, had been told that if I presented myself professionally and knowledgeably, the examiners would take this into account. He said the examiners weren't the slightest bit friendly and did nothing to make him feel comfortable. They had him in these little squares, about the size of a voting booth.

I couldn't help but wonder how much of what I was hearing was Dr. Cappucino's frustration. I had come too far to change my direction now. After dinner I decided to take a stroll by myself. Studying wouldn't do me much good at this point. I had a fight left. I convinced myself to be calm during the orals. Remember to be polite, confident, and not the slightest bit cocky. I still felt it was okay to say "I don't know." I would try to say what the examiner wanted to hear, no matter how farfetched.

I went back to my room and started studying the pathology atlas. I was most uncomfortable in this area and I knew I would see plenty of slides. I just prayed I would not get Dr. Cell. I had heard he was a coldhearted man and, unfortunately, Dr. Cappucino had run into this buzz saw. He was reputed by previous test takers to be the most likely to fail an applicant.

The next morning I purposely got up early so I could have breakfast by myself. I felt sorry for Dr. Cappucino but I wanted to be positive and I knew he would bring me down. After a last look at my notes, I was off to the ballroom. The instruction sheet on the door directed me to, you guessed it, pathology. Great. Just what I didn't need.

I got to my booth and was told to wait outside by the examiner, who was preparing the slides. But guess what? It wasn't Dr. Cell. That much I knew. This guy was much younger and actually looked friendly. He smiled at me when he told me to wait outside. Finally, the bell rang. I entered the booth and this rather boyish but large fellow stuck out his hand and said, "Good morning, Doctor. Please sit down and just relax." This wasn't so bad, yet.

He stated that he would present the history and physical examination of a patient, show me some x-rays, and then we would look at slides. After a brief history, he showed me the first case on x-ray. After seeing the x-ray, I had no idea what I was dealing with. It didn't look even vaguely familiar. I was trembling. When he asked me to look at the slide, I went from area to area and described what I saw. He made no comments while I was doing this. Then he asked me if I knew what the diagnosis was. I responded that I wasn't sure but I thought it was one of three diseases.

He smiled after I told him my differential diagnosis and simply went on to the next case. It was weird but he seemed content. We did three more cases, two of which I knew. Then the bell rang. It hadn't been that bad and he was pleasant. He gave me no clue as to how I had done, but he seemed impressed with the way I approached the slides and the manner in which I described the material. I left feeling the advice I had gotten was correct. He shook my hand again as I left.

The next two areas were fairly easy. There were general questions asked by reasonable people and I had no major difficulty. I felt I had conducted myself well and actually knew most of the cases. One was on children's orthopedics and the other on adult reconstruction. Both examiners seemed more focused on case management than on correct answers and I left both booths feeling that I passed.

I was ready for my final encounter. This was on trauma, where I should be best, because I had trained at a trauma hospital. One of my professors was a leading expert in the field. After this I was done. It would be over.

It was time for some showmanship and to have some fun. I entered the last booth and the examiner was a very elderly man with a large amount of dandruff on his black suit collar. He had a very thick accent as he said, "Good morning." My first case was a twenty-five-year-old male who had been riding a motorcycle and was hit by a car. "He presents to the emergency room with this x-ray and you are the ortho-pedic resident on call. How would you manage this case?" he asked.

I had waited a whole year for this case. My dreams had come true. He was trying to trick me. He wanted to see if I would act like an orthopedist and not like a doctor, jet this dude up to surgery and shove a rod down the fractured femur. But this treatment was unheard of when this old-timer trained fifty years ago. They treated everything conservatively and rarely operated. His generation was

trained that fractures were treated by casting or traction. My generation was trained to carry a knife.

"The first thing I would do is check to see that this patient's vital
signs are stable," I began. "Frequently these injuries involve a great
amount of blood loss. Once he was stabilized, I would explain that
there are several ways to treat this fracture, but that traction is safe
and you usually get a good result." I further explained that if problems developed or the alignment was bad, surgery might be a last
resort. My examiner smiled gently and seemed to love my explanation. I felt like I had just won an Oscar. I have never, and I mean
never, suggested that a patient with this type of fracture have traction. I must admit I had no clue where the traction equipment was
even kept in my hospital. It would have probably taken me over an
hour to rig it up.

What would I have really done in this emergency room situation?
I would have sent the medical student and the intern to see the
patient. After all the workup was done, I would have made an appearance and said as soon as an operating room was free, we would insert
a rod down the thigh bone and ship him out of the hospital in a few
days.

The final bell sounded and I shook his hand to leave. I knew the
orals had gone well, and if, by some chance, I passed the written, I
was home free. I hustled back to my room and called Dr. Cappucino.
He felt better about the written than the orals and we both agreed to
meet for a quick drink in the bar before we packed and headed to the
airport for our red-eye flight home.

On the bus ride back to the airport, we laughed about the last two
days and we both agreed that we had just faced the most demeaning
experience of our professional lives. But the die was cast. It was over.
There was nothing we could do about it now. We would have to wait
for three months and then the letter would arrive. As the time
approached, each day we asked each other, "Did you hear?" Three
months after the test, we heard. I passed. He failed.

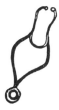

18. Bayview

I THOUGHT about leaving the Free For All Clinic, but where would I go? I recalled a conversation I had had during my residency with Dr. Islandia, an orthopedist in private practice. He was a funny man who was slightly aloof at times.

He loved to teach, so every week he drove 150 miles just so he could be with the residents in clinic and in surgery. Because of the long commute, he hired a pretty young girl to drive so he could spend time in the back seat dictating charts and filling out medical forms. He once told me, "When you get ready to go out into the real world and practice orthopedics, settle down where you want to live and where your wife will be happy."

One morning, Dr. Islandia came to assist us in surgery. We all changed into our scrub suits but then learned the case would be delayed about an hour. The chief resident, Dr. Hoppe, Dr. Islandia, and I decided to head down to the cafeteria for some coffee and a doughnut. Dr. Islandia was dressed for surgery in his booties, cap, and mask. Most of us put on the mask and hat just before entering the actual operating room. Many times doctors in the surgeons, lounge would stare at Dr. Islandia as he sipped a cup of coffee with his entire scrub suit in place.

We took the elevator all the way down to the cafeteria and people stared at Dr. Islandia with his mask on. Families thought they were in the midst of a robbery. As we entered the line in the cafeteria, my chief resident turned to me and said, "Listen, Buck, when do you think our leader is going to take off his costume? People are starting to look at us," he said angrily.

We tried to stay ahead of him in line to avoid too much embarrassment, but it was customary for the residents to buy doughnuts for the staff. Dr. Hoppe and I grabbed a doughnut and coffee and headed for the cashier's stand. The elderly cashier wasn't even slightly diplomatic as she peered through her bifocals at this amazing creature. By now our masked friend had captured the attention of the entire cafeteria. I quickly paid for all of us and strongly suggested we grab a table in the back corner.

Dr. Hoppe said I would be lucky if I ever got to do another surgical case this entire year. Jeez, all I did was suggest that we head down to the cafeteria for a quick snack. I watched in amazement as Dr. Islandia sat down, grabbed his doughnut, and attempted to take a bite of it through his mask. He chuckled at the unusual texture of his doughnut and then simply removed his mask and went on eating, as though the whole thing never happened. I peered back over my shoulder to count the number of my friends who would remind me of this day for the rest of my life.

It was Dr. Islandia who prompted me to start thinking about Bayview. I had enjoyed my first visit there nine years ago with my wife. It was the first time I met her parents. I was impressed with how cool the temperatures were in the morning. Her father, Cal, and I went out to play golf. He told me that Bayview was the greatest place in the world to live. I thought he had been smoking some of the funny stuff, because the newspapers frequently reported numerous murders, robberies, and demonstrations in Bayview. I could see the spectacular views and the weather were second to none, but the lifestyle and threat to personal safety concerned me.

I put on my best behavior for her dad. We teed off around 10:30 a.m. and the sun came out about 11:00. He belonged to a gorgeous country club, Piedmont Hills. The clubhouse was a magnificent Tudor mansion. The putting green surrounded a veranda. I thought if I ever moved to Bayview, I would join this club. I enjoyed the round on this short but challenging course, which was very narrow and well manicured. I was amused by my future father-in-law's right-wing political views. They were even further right than mine.

Cal and I had played golf again more recently and I mentioned that I would like to relocate to Bayview but that I knew nothing about orthopedic practice opportunities there. He said there was a member at the club, Dr. Quackmont, who was in sports medicine and, in fact, was the team physician for the local university. He asked me if I'd like to meet him and I said, "Great." He offered to arrange this soon. That afternoon, the weather remained delightful. A cool breeze filled the air as the sun set. This was my kind of weather. Golf weather. Twelve months a year.

A few days later, I gave Cal a call to thank him for the golf game. But I really wanted to know if he had touched base with Dr. Quackmont. He hadn't seen him at the club yet but offered to call him at home. I told him I was off again this weekend and would be willing to come down to Bayview if a meeting could be arranged. He returned my call that evening to say that Dr. Quackmont had suggested we meet for lunch at the club. I was ready to make my first serious attempt at finding a position outside the Free For All Clinic.

My wife and I arrived in Bayview around noon on Saturday. I dropped her off to visit her mom and I headed for the club in search of Cal and Dr. Quackmont. I found Cal sitting in front of his locker changing clothes. He said Dr. Quackmont was playing in the foursome right behind him and would be in shortly. We sat out on the veranda and waited.

Dr. Quackmont strolled over to our table. He was an elderly man, very pleasant, and receptive. "I understand from Cal that you're interested in sports medicine and want to practice in Bayview," he said. I agreed and told him a little of my background and present situation. He listened intensely and then described the environment in the local orthopedic community.

"There's one large group in the community that controls orthopedics. As a matter of fact, I went to college with Dr. Small, the head of the group. But over the past several years, many of the referring doctors in the community have wished for another orthopedist to whom they could refer patients. There are many doctors around who just don't like some of the personalities in the Small group," he said. He went on to explain, in confidence, of course, that there were some strange birds in this group.

He mentioned that Dr. Small was quite elderly and losing his surgical touch, and might even be interested in talking to me about a position in the group. But he suggested not joining them if I had any confidence in my ability to make it on my own.

He described Dr. Drab, the second-in-command of the Small group. He was unfriendly and marginally respected in the community. Then there was Dr. Pole, who did most of the total joint replacement in town. He was a good surgeon but rarely talked and frequently angered referring doctors by operating on their patients without telling them.

Another partner was Dr. Stalin. He was rude and abrasive not only with patients, but with many of the community doctors. He considered himself to be the arthroscopist of the universe but had no formal training in arthroscopy. Dr. Quackmont said it sounded like my experience was substantial compared to that of Dr. Stalin.

Dr. Quackmont finished by saying, "I could probably get you a spot in the group because of my relationship with Dr. Small. These guys have a corner on the market because there's no one else. They can treat people any way they please, and they do."

He mentioned there was another orthopedist in town, Dr. Laddie, but he was not busy. His partner was Dr. Ley, who was busier but very unpopular. Dr. Quackmont said Dr. Ley was very political in the community, and was having marital problems affecting the quality of his practice. Finally, there was Dr. Track, a young physician who was having trouble with privileges at the hospital.

I asked Dr. Quackmont what he would do. He suggested that I make an appointment to see both Dr. Small and Dr. Laddie and get their assessments of the community and how a new orthopedist might be received. He did offer me one ray of hope. He assured me that because of his position at the university, he could be very influential in getting me a job in the orthopedic department, even though this was run by Dr. Small. This would give me some business initially and some exposure to 35,000 students on campus, most of whom played intramural sports.

Dr. Quackmont had been incredibly helpful. I thanked him for all the information and for his advice. As he was leaving, I asked him if I could use his name in setting up these meetings and he insisted that I do. The three of us agreed to set up a golf game in two to three weeks.

As my father-in-law and I drove back to his house, he kept reiterating how influential Dr. Quackmont was in the community and at the university. If anyone could get me started in the community, it was

Dr. Quackmont. I felt good about the day and I sensed that I had a new lease on life. After dinner my wife and I headed back to Flatville.

I really believe in switching jobs or changing locations. I returned to the Free For All Clinic with a new outlook and charged into my little cubbyhole with a smile. I could see the brightly shining light at the end of the tunnel.

I decided to wait a few days to call Dr. Quackmont, as I didn't want to be annoying or overly aggressive. But I wanted to get to Bayview soon and I wasn't willing to be very patient. Dr. Quackmont called me three days later while I was in the clinic. After we exchanged the usual pleasantries and I thanked him again for taking the time to meet with me, he told me I had good timing. He said he had just received a call from Mr. Carnegie, the general manager and head football coach of the Bayview Intruders, a new professional football team that would be playing in the spring instead of the fall. I had heard of Mr. Carnegie and followed some of his teams in the college and professional ranks, but I knew little about the Spring Football League.

Dr. Quackmont said Mr. Carnegie had called to see if he was interested in being the team doctor for the Intruders. But when he learned that Dr. Quackmont was not an orthopedic surgeon, Mr. Carnegie had asked for a referral to another doctor in the area. Dr. Quackmont had said that I might be moving to the area. He asked if it was all right to give Mr. Carnegie my phone number. Is the sky blue? I told Dr. Quackmont how much I appreciated his confidence in me and that I anxiously awaited Mr. Carnegie's call. Dr. Quackmont said he would call him back immediately to tell him of my interest.

Never one to miss an opportunity, I asked if he had seen Dr. Small. He said he had talked with him in the coffee room yesterday. Dr. Small was interested in talking to me and he suggested that I call his secretary to set up an official appointment. Once again, I thanked Dr. Quackmont for his efforts on my behalf. I could hardly wait to call Dr. Small's office.

I returned to my patient and apologized for taking so long on the telephone. I felt particularly bad for this lady as she had been to four different physicians at the Free For All Clinic for knee pain. She was tired of getting the runaround, and here I was, on the phone for thirty minutes. She had hurt her knee in a softball game and felt a pop. She had gone to the emergency room, where the knee was splinted and she was given crutches. It didn't get better and she couldn't return to her job teaching school. Her family doctor told her to see me. My schedule was so full she was sent to Dr. Mumbles. He spent less than five minutes with her and told her she needed immediate surgery but never told her why. She grabbed her crutches and scampered out of his office.

Finally, she had gone to Dr. Done's office this morning. He called me to expedite the solution. After all, I owed him a favor. She had a classic presentation of torn cartilage so I snuck her onto the surgery schedule for the next day. She had a large tear in her cartilage which I removed the next morning in surgery. She went to her classroom two days later without her crutches.

The next day in clinic, I received the call. Jesus came over to the cast room as I was setting a wrist fracture and told me Mr. Carnegie was on my private line. My heart jumped. I asked the cast technician to hold this little girl's wrist while the cast dried and I bolted through the door to my office.

When I answered the phone a deep and distinguished voice roared, "Doctor, this is Jack Carnegie from the Bayview Intruders Football Team. I got your name from Dr. Quackmont, who said you were well trained and interested in sports medicine. He recommended you highly and I was wondering if you would like to be considered for the job?"

I told him I was very interested. Since it was Friday, I asked him if he would be around over the weekend and I would be happy to drive down to meet him. He was obviously impressed and said he would be in the office working on draft choices all weekend and to come at my convenience. I was delighted with this opportunity and this man. He sounded so charming and genuine, both unusual for a coach in professional sports. We talked briefly about my background and agreed to meet the next day around 10:00 a.m.

I was on a roll. I picked up the phone and called Dr. Small's secretary to see if I could arrange a meeting over the weekend. His secretary said he was in surgery but he would return my call before the end of the day. He never did. Was Dr. Quackmont telling me the truth about Dr. Small's interest in me?

Arriving at the Intruders' camp was exciting. There was a huge helmet logo on the door and it reminded me of my days with Dr. Rosey. I introduced myself to the pleasant-looking blond in the reception area who said she was expecting me and led me right back to Mr. Carnegie's office. She asked how my trip was from Flatville, like she knew about me already. We entered a large office in the back where a distinguished-looking man wearing an Intruders' jacket sat at a large desk.

He motioned for me to sit down as he spoke with someone on the phone about a player. His secretary brought me a cup of coffee and then Mr. Carnegie caught my attention when he told the other party on the phone, "Well, while you're deciding on my offer for your linebacker, I'm going to try to convince this young doctor in my office to become our team physician. Give me a call later. See you."

We both stood up as we smiled and shook hands. "Thank you for taking the time out of your busy schedule to make this long journey. I've heard many nice things about you from Dr. Quackmont. When are you going to relocate to this area?" he asked. We talked for about half an hour and I developed a sincere liking for this man.

I liked his philosophy. He didn't want a family physician for the team doctor because almost all player injuries were orthopedic. He agreed to let me bring other physicians around for consultation even though the team was willing to pay only me. I told him since I would be devoting a considerable amount of my time to the team and not to my practice, I would want a contract, just like the players. Also I would require my own team credit cards for expenses, such as supplies and travel. I wouldn't normally have been this demanding on my first interview but I could see he wanted me to take the job.

With little difficulty, we agreed to terms. I would be given a three-year contract at $30,000 per year, my own credit cards, and four complimentary seats to each game. I was happy because this income would be in addition to x-rays and surgeries performed on players and staff, for which there was additional insurance. Considering the liability, he agreed to pay for a malpractice policy. I had just established my base in Bayview. I had a salary, a following, and instant advertising at no charge. The team doctor had his picture in the team media guide as well as the weekly football magazine sold at the games.

I would be constantly quoted in the newspaper concerning player injuries. The bottom line was that Mr. Carnegie and I seemed to hit it off beautifully, as if we had known each other for years. I told him how excited I was to be involved with his team and with the new league. It was a new adventure, like moving to Bayview.

I think he was relieved that his doctor was already acquainted with professional football policies like injured reserve, preseason physicals, waivers, and player attitudes in general. How exciting for me. Finally, I was the team doctor, not under the wings of Dr. Rosey. I could call my own shots without answering to someone else.

Mr. Carnegie asked for my help in finding a trainer. He wanted to make the final decision, but if I could contact a few prospective applicants, he would be most appreciative. I agreed to get right on it and keep in close touch. I left feeling very good. I had a decent contract and, once I got down to Bayview, this would be a big feather in my cap. Who needed Dr. Small, anyway?

As I was heading out the door, Mr. Carnegie introduced me to the general manager. We entered a smoke-filled room where I met Mr. Polo, a pleasant, white-haired man with a red face. He immediately started joking about his bad back and how his very ill parents were here visiting from New Jersey. It would be great to have a doctor around, day and night, to help out in a crisis. Mr. Carnegie quickly briefed Mr. Polo about our financial agreement. Immediately Mr. Polo started kidding me how I'd better be damn good for that kind of money and give him all the free drugs he wanted. So you want to be a team doctor?

The last person I met before leaving the offices was the business manager, Mr. Leventhal. He worried me. He wanted to know my projected budget off the top of my head. "Well," I explained, "that's a tough one. But a few things that come to mind are the trainer and assistant trainer salaries, all the training equipment including tables, whirlpools, ultrasound, ice machines, and drugs." He sat down looking a little pale. He gingerly asked me if I had a rough estimate in dollars. I told him $200,000. My concern was that he looked like a fish out of water. He admitted he had never worked with a football team before and he only agreed to do this because he was a friend of the owner. However, he was starting to think this friendship might be drawing to a close.

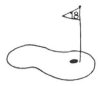

19. The First Fairway

WAS THIS a stroke of luck? As Cal, Dr. Quackmont, and I strolled down the first fairway and began the usual small talk, I started to calculate when I would ask Dr. Quackmont about my difficulty in reaching Dr. Small. I decided to wait until he hit a good shot so he'd be in a good mood. He finally did. It took four holes. It was a chip shot that landed two feet from the flag.

As we approached the green, he beat me to it and asked, "Have you given any more thought to your move down here?" I told him that I had made a firm commitment to myself to make the move and it was now only a matter of deciding where we would live and with which practice I would associate. I wanted him to be able to go back to Dr. Small and tell him, "This guy is really serious."

I felt this was the appropriate tactic for a very important reason. Often, when doctors hear that a new doctor is interested in coming to the community, they immediately see this as competition, and do everything in their power to discourage it. They pass the word around that it will be tough to get started in this tightly knit community and claim there are no more slots on the emergency room call schedule. They try to prevent the new doctor from getting hospital privileges. In general, they want to politely let the competition know, "keep the hell away."

However, if you state you are on your way to the community, they take a different stance. As long as he's coming, do we want this guy with us or against us? What if he is not with us and he gets real busy or the referring doctors like him more than us?

I told Dr. Quackmont, "I tried on two occasions to get through to Dr. Small and he never called me back. I have a tentative appointment with Dr. Laddie next Wednesday to see if he is interested in an association with me. Oh, and by the way, I did meet with Mr. Carnegie and things look good with the Bayview Intruders. I'm going to be the team doctor, and I want to thank you once again for your recommendation."

I could see that my statement distracted Dr. Quackmont. He missed the short putt after I sank my six-footer.

As we strolled over to the next tee area, he told me he couldn't understand why Dr. Small hadn't returned my call. He said that he had spoken to him just yesterday and Dr. Small sounded enthusiastic. The only problem was Dr. Ley, who had been in the community for several years and was also talking to Dr. Small about a position in the group. This got even more interesting because Dr. Ley was leaving Dr. Laddie, who had agreed to chat with me this week. Apparently Dr. Ley had a fairly busy practice, but a lot of physicians in the community thought he was abrupt and rude to patients and staff. Dr. Quackmont doubted that he would fit in well with Dr. Small's practice. He admitted, "I think if you come to town with your credentials and arthroscopy experience, and you are the team doctor for the Intruders, you'll be very busy in a hurry. Knowing Dr. Small, he won't want to risk not having you in his practice."

It seemed as though I had gotten my point across. He also told me that he worked part-time as a consultant at a physical therapy and sports medicine clinic and he frequently needed people to fill in there. So between my own practice, the Intruders, the sports medicine clinic, and the university privileges, I would be busy.

The rest of the round we talked football and golf. After we finished, Dr. Quackmont had a quick pop at the bar with us. As he left, he promised to speak with Dr. Small again on Monday morning and he would give me a call in the afternoon. I wasn't holding my breath, but Dr. Quackmont had been reliable and honest in the past. And he did get me the interview with Mr. Carnegie.

I had dinner with my wife and her parents. We talked seriously about the best areas to live in Bayview and which districts had the best schools. I felt this whole thing coming together and I was excited.

On Monday morning I decided to call Dr. Laddie and firm up our Wednesday meeting. I was interested in Dr. Ley's situation and why he was leaving Dr. Laddie. Dr. Laddie wasn't in but he returned my call an hour later. He said he would be around all afternoon on Wednesday and to stop by at my convenience. As far as Dr. Ley was concerned, he didn't sound too excited about talking over the phone, but he did say he would fill me in on the details on Wednesday.

My private line rang. It was Dr. Small, who said, "I'm sorry I haven't gotten back to you, but I've been extremely busy these past few weeks. I understand from Dr. Quackmont that you may be interested in practicing orthopedics in Bayview." He sounded worried.

I wondered if Dr. Quackmont had gotten through to him and what he might have said. "Yes, Dr. Small, I've made a firm commitment to relocate to Bayview. I've informed the Free For All Clinic that I would be leaving August first."

There was a noticeable silence. "Where have you decided to set up shop?" Dr. Small asked. I told him that I had spoken to a few doctors in the community and had given some consideration to opening an office on my own. He warned me that the community was locked up by his practice and that a move to Bayview would be a big mistake. I would be doomed to failure.

"But I would certainly like to meet you, especially since my good friend, Dr. Quackmont, has spoken so highly of you." He invited me to his office around lunchtime on Wednesday so we could talk. He promised to speak to his other partners so I could meet some of them too. I was annoyed that he had never called me back until now, and was calling out of fear. What did this new kid on the block have up his sleeve? I hadn't actually given formal notice to the Free For All Clinic, but everyone knew I had gone to Bayview on several occasions for interviews. These things leak out.

That afternoon while I was seeing patients, Dr. Mac came to my office wanting to know if I could spare a few minutes. Why hadn't I told him? Now I was in real trouble. "Buck, there are a few things I want to discuss with you and I feel bad that we haven't had more time to chat," he apologized. He looked a little peaked.

"First off, I'm a little miffed about this new arthroscopy equipment that the hospital has purchased for you. I wish you would come to me about these things. I know I haven't been very supportive of your specific arthroscopic needs, but the department has its priorities and when there are five people doing total joint surgery and only one doing arthroscopy, we go with the majority's needs first. Dr. Done told me that he gave you the money and asked me to be more supportive of you in the future. I have to think of the department first and not the individual people in it."

The same old song and dance. He wasn't really angry with me. What was he really after? "However, I know Dr. Done has already told you about your merit increase next month," he continued. "Both he and I are very pleased with your progress and the patients give you very high marks." I now knew where this was going. He wanted something. What it was became obvious when he commented, "There seems to be some clicking inside of my knee and I'm quite sure I have a torn cartilage. Do you think you might have a minute on your surgical schedule this week to take a peek inside with your new tools?"

I was flabbergasted. Dr. Mac wanted me to look inside his knee? "I'd be glad to scope your knee next week. Let's go down the hall and schedule it at a time convenient for you," I gleamed. We found him a slot, he thanked me, and off he limped.

I actually felt sorry for the man. He was a nice guy, but he had so much trouble expressing himself. I was getting the feeling he liked me, but I was too visible in the department and in the hospital. As chief, he didn't like that at all. I think he worried I would take over. But I wasn't even going to stay.

As I was getting ready to leave for the evening, Jesus asked me if he could have a word with me. What now? "Dr. Mays, I was wondering if you and your wife could come to my house for dinner on Friday night? You have done so much for me and I just wanted to thank you before you left the Free For All Clinic." I was startled. "Jesus, what makes you think I'm leaving?" I joked. He said that he figured with all the phone calls I had been receiving that the time was near. "Besides," he said, "no one who is good stays here for long." I told him I would be honored to come to his house and that I looked forward to it.

On Wednesday I arrived in Bayview early, so I stopped by to see Dr. Quackmont who was working in what had once been a funeral home. He seemed delighted to see me. As he showed me around the remodeled building, he asked about my agenda for the day. I told him that I had plans to see Dr. Small and his partners, and Dr. Laddie.

He motioned for me to step into his office and he shut the door. He said that Dr. Small had told him that Dr. Ley was negotiating to join his group. They were close to an agreement. Apparently Dr. Ley and Dr. Laddie were dissolving their partnership under fairly unpleasant circumstances. Dr. Quackmont admitted he wasn't excited to hear about this possible arrangement. He had gone so far as to tell Dr. Small that he should strongly consider me first. In any event, Dr. Quackmont promised to be supportive of me and to get the ball rolling quickly so I could obtain privileges at the university health center. I thanked him and headed for Dr. Small's office.

I arrived on time, but of course I had to sit in the waiting room for twenty minutes, wondering why I couldn't be sitting in his office. It seemed as though the die was cast anyway. His office manager finally escorted me into his consultation room. I sat and waited for another ten minutes before he finally entered.

I was amazed. Dr. Small stood four feet, seven inches tall. His wrinkled face looked as though he were eighty years old, but he had thick brown hair without a trace of gray. Then I realized it was dyed. He had the most insincere smile I had ever seen and he remarked how great it was that we had finally met. I had sent him a curriculum vitae, and he remarked that he had reviewed it and was impressed.

He immediately discussed the politics of the community and warned me that Bayview didn't have room for another orthopedic surgeon. He said he had spoken with his partners and they agreed that their practice didn't need another orthopedist. He further emphasized that they didn't have any more vacancies at the university health center but he would keep me in mind if I came to town.

This man was ice-cold and calculating. He was trying to scare me off. After fifteen minutes, he said there were several patients waiting, although the waiting room had been empty. He had arranged for Dr. Pole to see me and then I would have lunch with Dr. Stalin, the arthroscopist in the group.

I sat for another ten minutes in Dr. Pole's office, only to be told that he didn't see how a new orthopedist could make a living in the community and that their group was filled to capacity. He had no personality. Furthermore, their group had no interest in being associated with anyone working with a professional football team because the liability was far too great.

Then he had the nurse take me over to Dr. Stalin's office. He was no friendlier than his associates. He looked like a cobra and his eyes pierced through me like a laser. He informed me that even though I had fairly significant credentials, he did all the arthroscopy in Bayview and there wasn't enough for two people. He asked me why I wasn't a member of the World Arthroscopy Association with all my credentials. I told him I had never heard about it, but I would like to join. When I asked him if he would be interested in sponsoring me if I came to town, he responded, "It seems doubtful you'll come to Bayview. Wouldn't it be better to get a sponsor somewhere else when you finally decide where to practice?" He left for a few minutes to see one last patient and I tried to comprehend what was happening to me. Then I became angry. I realized I was being run out of town before I'd even arrived. He returned, grabbed his coat, and grudgingly invited me to join him for lunch.

In the hospital cafeteria, he made sure we grabbed a table in the corner, rather than sit with the rest of the medical community where he would be obligated to introduce me. He spent the entire lunch telling me how political the community had gotten. He said that Dr. Small's group had controlled Bayview for so long that several orthopedists had come and gone because the well had gone dry. He also volunteered another interesting bit of information: no one had ever gotten orthopedic privileges at the university unless they were in Dr. Small's office. He was amazed that Dr. Quackmont would even suggest that an outside physician apply for privileges at the university.

I asked him if he knew Dr. Ley and he nodded yes, but quickly changed the subject. When I asked if Dr. Ley was changing practices, he said he didn't know a thing about it. He made an attempt to get more involved in shop talk. He asked how I performed my lateral release operations for dislocating kneecaps through the arthroscope. I couldn't wait to get back to town to bury this Nazi!

20. Dr. Laddie and I

AS DR. STALIN and I finished what turned out to be a failed attempt on his part to discourage me, a tall, balding man walked up to our table. It was Dr. Laddie. Dr. Stalin begrudgingly introduced us. Dr. Laddie asked if he could join us and Dr. Stalin said he was just leaving. I had previously been told through the grapevine that Dr. Stalin was such an ass that when he was a resident one of his patients had stabbed him with a knife. I could see why.

Dr. Laddie seemed pleasant. He was a low-keyed gentleman with a great smile. He said he had at least an hour before office hours started and we might as well chat now instead of later. I agreed but wondered why he started his office hours at 2:30 in the afternoon. Sort of a long lunch hour, wouldn't you say? We started the conversation talking about golf, which was dear to both of us. It soon became apparent that Dr. Laddie was infatuated with the game and spent most of his time away from medicine playing golf. Dr. Quackmont had told me that it was well known throughout the community that Dr. Laddie was not readily available to answer emergency calls because he was usually on the golf course. Although he carried his beeper, he had no phone. This usually meant he would wait until the end of a round, sometimes two to three hours, before answering a page. This was only the tip of the iceberg, I would find out later.

I asked him about Dr. Ley's departure. He said how dreadful the whole thing had been. Dr. Ley was going through a bitter divorce and because Dr. Laddie and his wife had been close to Dr. Ley's wife over the years, Dr. Ley felt the need to abandon Dr. Laddie. "I don't know how much you've been told about the current situation around here, but Dr. Ley is joining Dr. Small's group and I am being left by myself," he muttered.

I found that fascinating. Especially since I had just spent time talking with Dr. Small, Dr. Pole, and Dr. Stalin, and none of them said a word except there was no more room in the community. Dr. Stalin had the gall to tell me he had no idea what Dr. Ley was doing and they had no more room in their group. Hey, this was going to be fun.

Dr. Laddie asked what was happening with the Intruders, as he had run into Dr. Quackmont a few days ago and he had mentioned I might be working with the team. I told him I had accepted the job and he looked excited. I asked if it would be possible to cover for me on the weekends I would be traveling with the team. He said he saw no problem with that and I offered to make up those call days during the off-season. It was funny how we were already talking about the office and he had not offered me a position and I had not asked to join him. But it was obvious. Neither of us cared for Dr. Small or his shabby group. I needed a place to hang my shingle and he needed someone to share the rent. Dr. Laddie said it was great that I had the Intruders as a means of getting started, since he wasn't sure how I was going to get any patients initially. At least until I had time to meet some of the physicians in the community.

I asked him if he received many referrals from the emergency room and he laughed. "What's so funny?" I inquired. "There is so much you don't know, Buck." He shook his head. He explained that I shouldn't expect to get any referrals out of the emergency room. He cited the frequent occasions he was sitting in his office while on call in the emergency room and Dr. Ley's secretary would come into the room to inform Dr. Ley that the emergency room nurse was on the phone for him. Dr. Laddie thought it was strange they were calling for Dr. Ley when Dr. Laddie was listed on-call. "For the longest time I could never understand it, but I just assumed he had more physician referrals than I, even though I had been in town twice as long as he had," he smiled.

The situation became painfully obvious over the next several months. Dr. Ley was having an affair with the head nurse in the emergency room. Of course she would direct all of the good cases with the best insurance to Dr. Ley, in spite of the call schedule, which was supposed to equally distribute emergency room patients to the community orthopedists. Dr. Laddie told me how the situation was even more pitifully close to home. He mentioned that on several mornings he had come into the office and found earrings on the couch in his consultation room. You guessed it. They belonged to Dr. Ley's squeeze from after-hour consultations.

I asked Dr. Laddie why he permitted this to go on. He stated he didn't know what he could do about the situation. It wasn't his style to rock the boat, even though he hadn't pinned a hip out of the emergency room for over six months. And furthermore, he said, he didn't want to mess with Dr. Ley's girlfriend, as she was the closest thing to a pit viper. She had the foulest mouth he had ever heard in a woman. I could hardly wait to sink my teeth into this under-the-table operation.

Dr. Laddie admitted that Dr. Ley's departure was the second medical breakup he had suffered and he wasn't willing to go through this again. I completely understood. I suggested that since he had extra space and I needed somewhere to go, I could rent half of the space from him and we could share supplies and x-ray expenses. Everything else could be separate. We would just associate. He agreed and asked me if I wanted to go over and take a look at the office and sit on the famous couch in his consultation room. I could hardly wait.

On the way over, Dr. Laddie told me he didn't think Dr. Ley's secretary, Nordy, was going to join Dr. Ley at Dr. Small's office. It seemed as though they didn't like each other much and she was looking for another job. Dr. Laddie thought she was a good secretary and that I might want to talk to her about working for me. It seemed like a good idea, but I wondered if it wouldn't look a little odd to the community, giving the impression that I had stolen Dr. Ley's secretary. We would see.

We entered the office and there were two people sitting at a small front desk. One was an elderly lady who looked me up and down. It was Dot, Dr. Laddie's secretary. I thanked her for helping me get through to Dr. Laddie on my numerous phone calls. She smiled. The other woman was very young and looked weathered and nervous. It was Nordy. As we all chatted, a chunky man appeared and gave me a sardonic look. It was Dr. Ley. "I heard you might be coming to Bayview," he said. I told him I was giving it serious consideration and

I was sure we would be seeing more of each other. He nodded and walked away.

Dr. Laddie showed me around the tiny office which was about eight hundred square feet, including two exam rooms, x-ray, a consultation room, and a waiting room. We finally settled in the consultation room as Dr. Ley walked out without saying good-bye or wishing me well. Dr. Laddie and I talked more about the arrangement and I was convinced he would be the best bet for me. Since I needed a friend in the community who wouldn't stab me in the back and a fairly small office that wouldn't cost me much money, I said I definitely wanted to join him and he agreed. I told him I would like to start the first of September and he approved. Dr. Ley would be gone by then, but not forgotten. As we spent a few minutes together laughing and trying to set up a golf game, I felt around the couch for more evidence.

I thanked Dr. Laddie for his time, told him I would be in touch, and how much I looked forward to an association with him. He agreed and I headed for the door. On my way across the street to the hospital, I noticed Nordy was sitting on the bench in front of the building. I figured this was no accident. I stopped to chat and she was quite delightful. I suggested we take a walk around the block in case Dr. Ley was spying on us. She laughed. In fact, what Dr. Laddie had said was true. She couldn't stand Dr. Ley and wanted another job. "Are you looking for a secretary?" she asked. I told her that I was and that I would be delighted to have her stay with me, but wouldn't it seem a little peculiar? She said, "Not really, since Dr. Ley is relocating to the other side of the hospital, which in reality is almost a totally different community." She said if it didn't bother me, it didn't bother her.

I told her it might be a little slow at first and I didn't know how I would keep her busy. But she said I didn't seem like the type to let any grass grow under my feet and since I was so interested in sports medicine, her husband might be able to help. She explained that he was the trainer at a nearby college and he might be able to send a few injuries my way. Great.

We chatted about Dr. Laddie for a while and Nordy told me I had made a good decision, because it appeared that Dr. Laddie and I would nicely complement each another. She said Dr. Laddie was very low-keyed and not the busiest orthopedist in town, but was very nice and easy to get along with. That's how it seemed to me, too. As we turned back toward the hospital, I asked Nordy if we had a deal and we shook hands. I told her she could start immediately when Dr. Ley departed, even if I had not arrived in Bayview. She agreed.

"Oh, by the way," I joked, "Dr. Laddie told me about the referrals Dr. Ley got through the emergency room on days he wasn't on call. Do you really believe this, or was Dr. Laddie exaggerating?" She smiled and looked at me like I had just won the lottery. She told me she had collected all the documents on these referrals over the last year and most of them were on days Dr. Ley was not on call. I could see that Nordy had no love lost for Dr. Ley and she appeared to want to get back at him. She told me she would make copies of the information after everyone had left the office and send me the evidence. I thanked her for everything and told her I thought we would make a great team.

She asked me if I would ever hit an employee. I was offended and asked her why. On two occasions Dr. Ley had struck her, and this was the main reason she could not tolerate him any longer. She was afraid of him. I assured her this was not my style and I wondered if he might not have done the same thing to his wife.

21. On Your Mark, Get Set, Go

THE STAGE was set. I was going to Bayview to set up shop. I would be associated with Dr. Laddie and we would butt heads with a five-man group of bandits. I couldn't help but laugh during my ride back to Flatville at the less than subtle attempts to bully me. Did they think they owned the community? I kept remembering that Dr. Quackmont had told me how poorly liked this group was but they were the only game in town, so far.

The next day at the Free For All Clinic I wondered how I would break the news to everyone. But they got to me first. When I reached my desk, there was a note telling me to contact Dr. Done in his office, immediately. I made rounds on my patients and then stopped by his office before clinic.

He was sitting at his desk frantically puffing on his pipe. I could barely see through the haze. He looked irritated. "Come in and close the door, Buck," he ordered. "I've been hearing rumors around the hospital that you may be leaving us. Is that true?" I explained to him that, even though I was happy at the Free For All Clinic and had gotten a wealth of experience, I had always wanted to be in private practice on my own and I had a good opportunity to go to Bayview. I reiterated how much I appreciated his support and I was sure he would find another orthopedist to take my place.

"What's it going to take to get you to stay, Doc?" he asked as he bolted from his chair and started walking around the room. I tried to explain that I was ready to return to private practice at this stage of my career and now that I was the team doctor for the Intruders, it only made sense to be closer to the team.

I told Dr. Done that I could never be happy on a continuing basis at the Free For All Clinic unless I was chief of the orthopedic department and earning at least three to four times my present salary. He agreed that the salary would never improve to that level for even the highest-paid physician and that the head of the department would not change for at least three years. As I got up to leave, I could see he was disappointed.

He liked me and my style because I had spunk in a department filled with deadbeats. I asked him not to say anything to Dr. Mac since I wanted to tell him directly. It was, after all, the right way. The only way.

That same afternoon, after clinic, I told Dr. Mac. He merely responded that he'd always known I was a short-termer and that I would be better off in private practice with all my energy. I wasn't sure if he meant that as a compliment because I knew my energy level had constantly been a thorn in his side and considerable jealousy had developed between us. After all, I was more popular than he and I was three times busier.

He was totally ineffective at running the orthopedic department and I often reminded him of that fact at our weekly conferences. Although we got along okay, he knew I was always looking over his shoulder. If I needed something, I went to Dr. Done and this annoyed him tremendously. He took the news in stride and wished me luck. After all, I was still scheduled to operate on him next week and he didn't want me to accidentally leave a sponge in his knee.

The news spread like wildfire. I was inundated with calls from people in every department. They wanted to know the story behind my departure. All this fuss made me feel wanted, but my goal was to just keep the peace, so I told anyone interested that I was merely moving along to greener pastures and I appreciated the support and confidence of the staff. I began telling all the nurses I was booking no more surgeries but I would complete everyone I had scheduled. I felt it was inappropriate to operate on people and not be available for postoperative care.

Friday night my wife and I went to Jesus' house for dinner as planned. Jesus must have invited every relative in the county. There were at least thirty people at his house. It was a huge celebration of some sort. As I had a chance to go around and meet everyone, it became clear that several people had traveled over two hundred miles to get there.

After an incredible Mexican feast, Jesus stood at the head of the table and asked for quiet. "I want to thank everyone for coming tonight because I wanted you to meet my boss, Dr. Mays, before he leaves the Free For All Clinic. As most of you know, I have had a few ups and a lot of downs in my life. I didn't finish school and have had my scrapes with the law. I've worked at the clinic for ten years and have been transferred to a different part of the hospital every few months. Everyone thought I was stupid. I hated it, but it was a job.

"Then Dr. Mays showed up. The new guy on the block. The entire hospital laughed behind his back when I was assigned to him. But Dr. Mays was different. I could see it right from the start. He called me by my name instead of 'Hey you' and told me the first day that if I kept up with him, and was nice to his patients, we would make a great team. When he mentioned me to his patients he referred to me as his nurse, not his assistant. He taught me how to put on casts and take out stitches while all of the other doctors had continually told me I was a liability and poorly trained for my position.

"One previous doctor had told me I should switch to being a janitor. Dr. Mays even let me assist in surgery when they were short-handed and taught me how to hold retractors and cut knots. So I just wanted to say, Dr. Mays, that after forty years of my life, you made me feel like a human being who was needed and respected, and I wanted my whole family to meet you before you leave. Thank you for giving me some self-respect. I will never forget you."

I was teary-eyed and embarrassed as the entire throng stood up and clapped. After I wiped my face and my nose, I stood up to respond, trying to figure out how I could possibly top that. I looked around the table, trying to gain my composure, and all of these smiling faces stared at me. I began, "I must confess that on my first day at the clinic, when I was introduced to Jesus as my assistant, I said to myself, Oh shit! Here was this little Mexican in white pants, staring at me through glasses that had to be at least an inch thick. But he was nice, had a smile on his face, and I liked his attitude. He seemed intent on pleasing me. He said he was excited to be with a new doctor and would try to learn all the things I liked, and if I gave him a chance, he would be the best. He apologized for anything negative I might have heard about him from anyone else."

I paused, looked around the room, and by now, everyone had tears in their eyes, including my wife. I continued, "One of the things I've always done in my life, sometimes to my detriment, is to root for the underdog. I loved rooting for you, Jesus. And you know what, you clearly became the best nurse in the department over a short period of time. Dr. Mac even admitted you had made a complete turn-around. You were asked to help him on days when I was gone and he was short-staffed. His nursing supervisor came to me and told me whatever I had done, a new fire had been lit under Jesus and she was thrilled. Yes, you have done it all. I like your style. You don't brag or talk, you just continue to improve."

I giggled, "You remember, Jesus, the day in clinic when I had a head lock on that screaming child that needed suturing. The mother couldn't stand all the noise, so when she left, I told you to quick put in two sutures. I barely got the words out of my mouth, when you placed two sutures into the kid's arm like you had done it ten times before. That's because you knew more than everyone thought. You saw more than anyone realized. The final blow came when the mother returned, and I explained that as soon as I could put the cast on the arm, the little guy could go home. She said, 'Not to worry, because Jesus can cast the arm. He does a good job.' I knew that." I ended up saying how touched I was to be honored by such a large and warm family and how grateful I felt to have Jesus as my nurse.

That party turned out to be the start of my farewells. Plans progressed rapidly toward my move to Bayview and I quickly closed out my practice at the Free For All Clinic. We put our house on the market and I couldn't help but ask myself if I was doing the right thing. Would I be able to make it in a new and hostile setting? Was I being irresponsible to my family?

People invited me over for dinner and it seemed like I was going out to lunch daily with staff physicians saying good-bye. I spoke to Dr. Quackmont on several occasions and he continually encouraged me that I had made the right decision. He reiterated that I would be too stymied in Dr. Small's office. Again, as in the past, he vowed that he would do everything in his power to help me gain privileges at the university and he would send me athletic injuries from his practice.

The surgery went fine on Dr. Mac's knee. There was a small tear in his cartilage that was easily fixed and some minor arthritic changes on the end of his bone. All in all, he did beautifully. He made me look very good by stopping by the office the day after surgery to get his messages. He hardly had a limp. I could see, in his noncommittal way, he was impressed with arthroscopy. I'm sure he was feeling embarrassed as he recalled the trouble he had given me when I first came to the Free For All Clinic. Too bad he didn't appreciate it sooner, but it still meant something to me. I had proved my point.

One potential hassle was surfacing on my application to Bayview General because of some nasty comments made about me to the credentials committee by Drs. Cataract and Round of Flatville. Dr. Cataract had written that my privileges had been suspended at a local hospital because I was too aggressive as a surgeon. What he didn't say was that the emergency room doctors had been so much more impressed with my skills than his that he received no more referrals from the emergency room.

Dr. Round had written to the committee that I was very money-oriented. That resulted from my questioning him after he paid me one-fourth of my promised salary for covering his practice. He said, "Regardless of what I promised him, the money I paid him was enough for a guy just starting." What actually happened to all of the money he billed for my extensive services while he was on vacation? Seemingly, it was used to pay off multiple debts he had accumulated because his secretaries had not billed for any services in over six months.

I spoke to Dr. Writer, the chairman of the credentials committee at Bayview. He said that he doubted there would be a problem, but he had to follow through on these letters. I began to be alarmed at the thought I might not get privileges. I had told everyone that I had quit the Free For All Clinic. I started to wonder if Dr. Small had infiltrated the credentialing process, but Dr. Writer assured me he didn't really care for Dr. Small or what he had to say. Fortunately, in about a week, Dr. Writer called to say I had been granted temporary privileges. He laughed and stated, "You sure have a bunch of jealous orthopedists up in Flatville. No matter how many I spoke to, none of them had anything bad to say about you, only that you were very busy for a guy just starting practice."

In another three weeks, I quit the Free For All Clinic. Now my two concerns were the Intruders and the move to Bayview. The primary focus was on the Intruders. Since this was a league that played in the spring, the training camp was in the winter. Luckily the camp was in beautiful Arizona. Every week for six weeks, I journeyed to the desert to set up the medical team. This involved trainers, equipment, protocols for physical examinations, and medicines that would be required both at the training camp and in our traveling bags. I gave physicals to the players and examined injuries that didn't respond to treatment by the trainers.

This turned out to be a large time commitment, much greater than being an orthopedic consultant with Dr. Rosey. But it was fun and exciting, a new league with new people and a new challenge. This was in addition to my other new challenge, getting ready to step into a community where the competition was fierce and at least five guys wanted to see me dead.

I started going to Arizona while I was still at the Free For All Clinic. This set up a very unusual set of circumstances, to say the least. But it illustrates what you can do if you're determined. Here I was, still practicing in Flatville, while being the team doctor for a professional football team one hundred miles away. People read with amazement and curiosity when the paper reported that the starting tackle for the Bayview Intruders suffered a serious knee injury in Arizona and was flown to Flatville for surgery. The people in Bayview were the most confused, not to mention the players. But the staff, physicians, and administration at the Free For All Clinic were glad to have this free publicity.

The local newspaper ran several articles about me and the clinic. Of course the public relations office for the Free For All Clinic was very cooperative because this advertising was free. I didn't mind because I felt I owed something to the hospital.

The physicians would bring their kids by the players' rooms after surgery and the team donated shirts and pennants as giveaways. Other patients would just hang around my office hoping to get a glimpse of a real, live professional football player.

I had one final surgical hurrah at the clinic. A famous coach at the university in Bayview brought his wife to see me on referral from Dr. Quackmont. She was a professional dancer who noticed her left thigh didn't fit into her tight jeans anymore. Her right leg fit fine. Bad news. It was a tumor in the muscle of the thigh, which we removed through an incision that went from her buttock crease to the back of her knee. As a friend of the patient, Dr. Quackmont drove to Flatville and assisted me in surgery. The patient did well with some therapy and aggressive rehabilitation and danced again in a few months. Dr. Quackmont spread the word of our surgical triumph to the medical staff at Bayview, which I'm sure was halitosis to Dr. Small.

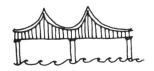

22. Bayview Boogie

MOST of the remainder of the summer I spent commuting to the Intruders' training camp outside Bayview. I spent two months doing mostly football. I devoted little time to setting up my practice, which I intended to start in full swing during the late summer. I frequently stayed overnight at my in-laws' house in Bayview because my daily commute was one hundred miles in each direction. This didn't enhance life with my wife and kids, but I reasoned that the investment in the football team would go a long way toward establishing me and my reputation in Bayview. It produced a good financial foundation.

The first year with the Intruders was a fascinating experience for me because it was totally different from what I had gone through with Dr. Rosey. With the Intruders, I was in charge and made all the decisions. With Dr. Rosey, I had been his assistant. I didn't have to make many decisions, and I didn't have to deal directly with the owner or management.

Before the season started, I had a meeting with Mr. Kent, the attorney for the Intruders and a close friend of the owner, Mr. Twitch. This meeting was a very memorable one, as we met for lunch at a restaurant on the bay. He showed up forty minutes late. I had been eager to leave, but I didn't want our relationship to get off on the wrong foot, so I impatiently waited until he arrived. I would come to realize over the next several months that this was the norm for Mr. Kent. But he was a pleasant man and I liked his approach to my relationship with the Intruders.

He agreed that since I would be spending so much time with the team, which was time out of my medical practice, I should have a contract. This new league seemed to have substantial financial backing, but what if it failed? At least I would have a contract to fall back on.

I thought it was very strange that Mr. Kent ordered no lunch, just a glass of milk. I kept offering him half of my sandwich, but he insisted he wasn't hungry although he kept picking up crumbs off my plate. He had absolutely no reason not to eat as he was as skinny as a rail. I could see why.

He finalized the details that Mr. Carnegie and I had agreed upon. I didn't ask for much, but I made sure everything I wanted was clearly stated in the contract. Between my salary and the office visits and surgeries, I figured I would earn over $50,000 a year from the team alone. I got my own credit card for travel in case of emergency when I couldn't fly with the team.

He agreed without much discussion. However, because I was the team doctor, he said I was expected to travel with the club during all away games and I agreed. Lastly, I insisted I have my own room on the road and at training camp prior to the season. I liked privacy and, more importantly, players would come to my room to talk about problems or injuries and I thought it more appropriate that I be alone. He agreed.

The first year of this spring league was pleasurable. The quality of play, as expected, was not that of the men in the fall, but a close second, and there was plenty of excitement. As I stood on the sidelines during the games, I realized many of the players would fit in well in any professional league. The first home game was memorable because we came from behind to tie the game in the last few seconds. We had the momentum and it appeared as though we would win. What a great start that would be, and it would bring fans back to the next game.

It also was reminiscent of a local team in the past which had earned a reputation for coming from behind and winning. The stage was set. No better script could have been written. Most of the fans in the stands had showed up just to see what this new league was all about. They were excited. It was just like old times. But we lost. Our kicker missed a field goal that my grandmother could have kicked. It was devastating. The fans piled out of the park thinking this was a poor substitute for the real thing.

But the team improved and we started winning games, not only at home but on the road. We remained in the top of the standings all season. The traveling was tough on the players, but convenient for me. We traveled to away games on Saturday for Sunday games, no matter how far away they were. If we left on Friday, like the teams in the fall, it would have cost another night of hotel lodgings and meals, and the owner wanted to keep costs down.

But what he didn't understand was that a player who traveled across country needed to adjust to the time zone difference. Arriving late Saturday night for a Sunday morning game was too tough and the players didn't play well. If the players didn't play well, the team lost more and they wouldn't make the playoffs. Then the team wouldn't get playoff money from the league. So it was a two-edged sword. I knew all this, but no one asked my opinion, so I kept quiet. I got to spend Fridays in my office and this was a bonus for my practice.

My responsibilities as the team physician were variable and interesting, as you might imagine. Yes, there were the obvious duties of taking care of the players. But there were many more obligations than that. At the preseason training camp in Arizona, I had to give all the players a physical examination and, of course, not everyone passed. There were many reasons for failing. Sometimes a past medical history endangered a player, like an old neck injury which caused repeated fainting spells on the field. Some had significant records of drug abuse.

One part of the job that I considered unpleasant and dangerous was the so-called departure physical. This had to be done when a player was cut from the team, or waived, or, for whatever reason, wasn't wanted by the coach or the management. These physicals were given to the departing players to ensure that they were healthy when they left the team, so the player couldn't sue the team.

One evening, a few days before we were to break preseason camp, the trainer and I were informed that all the coaches would be meeting to compile the final list of players who would make the team and those that would be cut. Mr. Carnegie told me that I would be furnished with the list of departing players. First thing in the morning, one of the coaches would go to the rooms of the cut players to tell them the bad news.

In professional football circles, this lucky coach was called the

Turk. The trainer and I were to follow immediately behind so we could give the physical before the incensed player bolted out the door and headed for the airport. Some of the players knew they weren't making the grade, but others would find the news a real shock. Most importantly, I didn't want them taking out their anger on me.

I was less than excited about this part of the job. I was going to knock on the door of some three-hundred-pound tackle who had just been told by a coach that his dreams of playing professional football were over. The guy might shoot the next person who knocked on the door. What if he refused to have the physical and wouldn't sign the release? I wasn't going to force him. I'd tell him that according to league rules, he needed a departing physical so he'd be eligible to sign with another team. Brilliant!

The trainer and I got up the next morning and had breakfast with the team. The atmosphere in the room was noticeably and understandably different than it had been on earlier days in camp. Very few players were talking to each other. The usually noisy room with everyone telling jokes and old football stories was pathologically quiet. Everybody knew what was coming down.

Then Coach Carnegie got up to speak. "Listen up, fellows. As you all know, today is the final day to trim our rosters. We hope that those of you who don't make the squad will not take the news personally. We feel each and every one of you is an excellent football player and every man in this room can find a spot on some club in the league. Please cooperate with us by returning to your rooms now so that Coach Lanyurt can come by and tell you of your status. If you make the team, he will be giving you a schedule for the rest of the week. If you don't make the team, you must have a physical before you leave. The trainer and doctor will come by to do that. If you want to waive your right to have a physical, you can simply sign a form saying so. Good luck to all of you men and God bless you."

As the players filed out of the room, I looked around and began to speculate which players I would be seeing shortly. Coach Carnegie came to our table and handed us the list of players to be cut. He jokingly said he was glad he wasn't in our shoes and, with a giggle, turned around and left. We sat there for ten minutes and mapped out the path we would take in the large hotel complex. We both agreed we should give the Turk a few extra minutes to get his job done.

I grabbed the necessary forms, my doctor's bag, and we headed out on our mission. Approaching the first room, we were relieved to see the door was already open. Our first prey was lying on the floor doing his stretching exercises so we walked in. The trainer said, "Hey, what's doing, big guy?" This big black tight end stood up and asked what we wanted. The trainer answered, "We need to do your physical before you leave." I stepped back when the player's face grew angry. He turned and walked away. Then he shouted, "Does this mean I'm cut? This team is the lowest organization I've ever been with. They send around the trainer and doctor to give us the bad news. What's the matter? Are those crappy coaches too chicken to face us themselves?"

The trainer and I looked at each other, puzzled that the coach hadn't been there before us. I quickly tried to recall what my wife always said when she crossed herself. "Where do I sign? I don't want your dumb physical," he yelled. "I'll waive the physical like you assholes are waiving me."

After he scribbled his name across the sheet of paper, the trainer and I headed back to Coach Carnegie's room under a head of steam. When he wasn't there, we headed to the breakfast area to see if he was still eating. We arrived to see him and the Turk at the table. "What the hell are you doing here? I thought you were going to get to the rooms before we did and inform those players that were cut? The doc and I have been out there doing your dirty work," the trainer yelled. Coach Carnegie looked at him in disgust and the Turk replied, "Hey guys, it's no big deal. I was just on my way out the door." We shook our heads in disbelief as he left the room, and the coach suggested he should have given this task to someone else. The trainer and I agreed we had done our last favor for him. Let him suffer if he ever needs our remedies.

We waited about twenty minutes before embarking on our mission again. The rest of the morning went without another blowup. I had grown close to some of the players cut, even if they didn't stand out on the football field. Each player had his own personality and several of them were funny and sensitive. Many signed the forms without incident. Some said that they were injured at camp and wouldn't sign or permit a physical. They assured us their attorneys would be in touch. Some were already gone when we got to their rooms.

During the first year, we traveled across the country and had several memorable experiences. We played in a virtual typhoon in New England. I had never been in rain and wind of that magnitude. But we ended up winning the game.

During that game the quarterback, Yuba, was tackled hard on a passing play and landed on his throwing shoulder. The trainer and I charged onto the field. After a minute of reassuring him that the shoulder was not broken, we helped him to the sideline and sat him on the bench.

As I was feeling under his shoulder pads to find out whether his shoulder was sprained, separated, or dislocated, I could see Coach Carnegie heading in my direction. He clearly was the most positive thinker I had ever encountered in my life. "Hey Doc, is he ready to get back in the huddle?" he begged. I told him that it looked like a minor shoulder separation and to send in the backup quarterback for at least a few plays.

Our victim thanked me profusely and I told him to take a few minutes to relax. He was obviously in a great deal of pain. But I reassured him that the shoulder was not seriously injured and he'd be okay. The second-string quarterback did a rather poor job filling in and so we punted the ball and the defense took over. I knew this would not please Coach Carnegie in this close game. We needed to win.

Five minutes later our defense held nicely and the other team punted. Coach Carnegie came over and smiled, "Hey Yuba, how's the shoulder?" He answered that it was sore. But the coach handed him a ball and demanded, "Let's see you throw one." I mumbled that I thought we should give him a little longer as Yuba stood up and shot-putted the ball about four feet. He winced in pain. "Hey, Yuba, I've never seen you throw the ball better. Get back in there," the coach yelled. I couldn't believe what was happening. Yuba charged back onto the field.

Fortunately, the field and the ball were so wet almost all of the downs were running plays, so he merely had to hand the ball off to one of the running backs. We were moving the ball well. We won. After the game, we were all grateful to be in the locker room, out of the rain, and that there were no major injuries. Yuba had a mild separation and the x-rays were normal.

The plane ride home was always much easier after a win. Everybody felt fine after a win. After a loss, everybody hurt and wanted pills.

Another task of the team physician, not previously explained to me, was bed check. Coach Carnegie felt that the doctor and the trainer should always do bed check in case one of the players wasn't feeling well or needed a sleeping pill or some aspirin. And, of course, bed check meant making sure all of the players were in their rooms by the designated curfew. Some of the trainers and previous coaches I had worked with made the rounds with the hotel security guard, who just blasted into each room.

I preferred to knock on each player's door, one by one. This meant that even if a player was asleep, he had to get up to open his door. I learned you never took anyone's word for it. You had to see the whites of their eyes. Most of the time, though, the players were in their rooms watching television or talking on the phone. Once in a while you would even find one studying his play book.

Sometimes you had to look a little closer at the situation. Players liked to cover up for each other. Like the time I waited a good five minutes for a player to come to the door. He appeared sleepy-eyed and tired and when I peered into the room, his roommate looked comfortably tucked under the covers. I said goodnight and went on to the next room. Just then, the player I thought was tucked away galloped past me in the hallway gasping, "I'll be in bed in thirty seconds. Please don't tell the coach, Doc." The old pillow trick had fooled me again.

In these cases, I really felt torn. If I told the coach, he might suspend the player. This was our star running back. If he didn't play, and the team lost, we would have an incredibly long flight home, and everyone would be pissed off the entire next week because we had been beaten. What would you do? I had a tendency not to squeal.

But I learned quickly. Once the trainer and I were approaching the last room of bed check, and it sounded like a party was going on. We knocked on the door and immediately there was total silence. We looked at each other with suspicion. After several minutes, the door opened. Yet another sleepy face answered the door and yawned. The lights were out and the player assured us they were both sound asleep.

But what the hell do these jokers take us for? We entered the room and turned the lights on. The other player sat up in bed and asked, "Hey, what you all think you're doing? I was sound asleep. Wait 'til I tell the coach you interrupted my beauty sleep when I miss those blocks in the game tomorrow." I started to feel guilty, as the room was mysteriously quiet and not a creature was stirring. We apologized and headed for the door.

But damn it, what was all that noise we'd heard? I told the trainer to wait a second. I entered the bathroom and turned on the light. I heard a faint giggle. I yanked open the shower curtain to find four pretty girls, minimally clothed, hiding in the bathtub. "Hey Doc, I don't have any idea how they got there. They must have snuck in, waiting for us to go to sleep so they could steal our jewelry," shouted one of the guys.

The team doctor also had other folks to take care of, like the cheer-leaders. At one game, I was summoned by the choreographer because one of his cheerleaders had fallen down, twisting her ankle. She was sitting on the ground in tears with an ice pack on her ankle. She was tall, thin, blond, and beautiful.

I introduced myself and took a look at this very swollen ankle. The rest of the cheerleaders were out on the field performing as I looked around for another body to help me get her into the locker room for an x-ray. I suggested she put her arm around me and we would make our way back to x-ray to see if anything was broken.

We stopped halfway there and she apologized for holding onto me too tightly, but I told her, "Hey, this is my job." I said "If nothing is broken, we can tape up the ankle for you, and you can get back out on the field." I told her I had considerably more training on taping ankles than the trainer. (I think I had taped one ankle in the last two years, and that was on the team photographer.) As we approached the x-ray room, she grabbed on tighter as the foot became more uncomfortable. Her large breast was pressing against my face. I strained to keep my composure.

When we arrived, the x-ray technician looked up from reading the day's program and leaped out of his chair, almost severing his nose on the x-ray machine. He took a quick film and there were no broken bones, so our glamorous patient hopped next door to the training room. I grabbed her thigh to help her onto the training table so I could tape her ankle.

One of the assistant trainers, in the room cleaning up, saw me stumbling around for some tape. "Can I tape the lady up for you, Doc?" he begged. "This is a pretty bad sprain, Jimmy," I responded.

"I better do this one myself," I answered, refusing to look him in the eye. I quickly refreshed my memory on ankle taping and wrapped her up, probably higher than I needed to go. Then I fitted her for some crutches. Once again Jimmy offered to assist, but I told him these particular crutches were very hard to adjust and I had better do it myself. After I allowed him to wrap an ice bag around her ankle, we headed back onto the field as her colleagues cheered her return. She agreed to come to my office in a few days so I could put her in a walking cast. It was a dirty job, but someone had to do it.

The people on and around the field were only a part of my responsibilities as the team physician. I received a call in my office one day from June, who was the new executive assistant to the vice president of the team. "Hi, Dr. Mays, this is June in the Intruders' office. I'm sorry to trouble you, but I didn't know who else to call and I need a favor. As you know, I just started working here and I haven't had time to find a doctor yet. Anyway, I wonder if you could call in a prescription for a new diaphragm for me?"

There was complete silence. "Dr. Mays, are you there?" she asked. Gaining my composure, I tried to think of something intelligent to say. "As you know, June, I'm an orthopedic surgeon and I don't normally do diaphragms," I whimpered. "I mean, I don't even remember anything about them other than that they come in sizes, don't they? Perhaps you should call a gynecologist. I'd be happy to refer you to one," I promised. "Dr. Mays, that would be fine under normal circumstances. But I don't think you understand, I need a new one by this evening," she pleaded.

I was starting to catch on. "Okay, June, I'll do it this one time but if it's the wrong size and you get pregnant, don't blame me," I said. "By the way, what size fits you?" She replied, "You know, Dr. Mays, I've forgotten, so hold on one second while I check!" My head sunk in my hands. "Thanks for waiting, Dr. Mays. It looks like a size seven but the number has been worn away," she said.

I told June I would call the team pharmacy to order it. She thanked me and said she owed me one. No thanks. I was trying to figure out how I could call the team pharmacist and still save face. No way. He would laugh me out of town. I know. I'll have my secretary call. But I couldn't do that, either. She would be suspicious.

I grabbed the phone book and found a pharmacy near our team

office. When the pharmacist answered the phone, I tried to be very much in control, "Hi, this is Dr. Mays calling from Bayview for a prescription for a June Lovell. She needs a number seven diaphragm." I did it and I was very convincing on top of it. He bought the whole thing. I could hear him repeating my order as he was writing. Slam dunk.

He muttered, "Yes, Dr. Mays, and what brand did you want her to have?" Oh shit! What brand? How do I know what brand? What a stupid question. "Oh gee, I don't know, what's a good one?" I asked. I heard laughter. My cover was blown. "I'm sorry for laughing, Dr. Mays, but are you an OB/GYN man?" he chuckled. I figured at this point, what the hell. I may as well tell him the entire story so he could get a laugh out of it too. And he did. He roared. Then he sympathized with me and told me the most common brand and I said, "Go for it."

We chatted for a spell about football and the Intruders. He said he was a fan and that some of the players had been in his store. I told him I would send him four seats to the next game and thanked him for his understanding and hung up. I immediately called June and told her where to pick up the goods and to make sure she took the pharmacist four good complimentary seats to the next game.

As I was leaving my office that evening, my secretary said, "Oh, I almost forgot to tell you. A Mr. Louie called you from the Good Times Pharmacy to thank you for the tickets to the game. He said he hoped you guys could do business again soon." She turned away with a smirk on her face.

23. Present the Lineups

I WAS ready to start the game. I envisioned the two teams presenting their lineups to the umpires at home plate. The stage was set. It was Dr. Laddie and I against Dr. Small and his misfits. But that was okay. I always liked good, clean competition. I had no idea how dirty the opposition would get.

My first day I set out as Dr. Laddie had suggested. Meet as many people as I could and spend at least thirty minutes each morning in the doctors' coffee room at the hospital to meet members of the medical staff. The more I hung around the more likely I would run into another doctor who just might say, "Hey, would you like to see a patient for me?"

I arrived in the coffee room at 7:30 a.m. sharp, but to my surprise it was empty. So I grabbed a cup of coffee and sat down to read the sports page. Within five minutes Dr. Small came walking in, recognized me immediately, and somewhat begrudgingly stuck out his hand. "When did you start?" he questioned. "This is my first day, so I thought I'd come to the coffee room and see if I could meet some of the staff," I answered. He wandered toward the doughnuts and, without looking at me, muttered, "Well, it's just like I told you when you came to my office, this community doesn't need another orthopedic surgeon."

I felt a rush come over my entire body. I had been in the community less than ten minutes and already my competition had told me I wasn't welcome. But in retrospect, it was just the stimulus I needed. It was then that I vowed to bury him.

He asked me exactly how Dr. Laddie and I were set up in practice. I told him that had not been decided, although it obviously had. I was impressed at how quickly this midget got nosy.

I met several people in the coffee room that morning and I made sure to introduce myself to everyone, even though some seemed unfriendly. My message to all was the same. I'm new in town, I have no patients, and I'm available twenty-four hours a day, seven days a week. If you need a bone setter for any type of patient, young or old, good insurance or bad, call me.

There were a few doctors who made a lasting impression on me that morning. Dr. Feldman was an elderly internist. He worked in the same building as I did and his message to me was clear. He was "the professor" in this town and if he liked a young man who was new, he would send him lots of work and help him establish a practice. He pointed his finger at me on several occasions and lectured me about starting out. I simply nodded each time and agreed. After all, if he had the patients, I had the time to listen, all day, every day. He told me that his practice consisted mostly of faculty at the local university. His history was even more interesting. He explained he was Jewish and when he first came to town, the doctors wouldn't let him on the medical staff at Bayview. He had had to skimp and struggle for patients some thirty-five years ago.

He said I would do well if I followed the three A's: appearance, ability, and availability, and not necessarily in that order. I felt very positive about this man, and told myself if I could tolerate his talking down to me, I could get business from him. That was what I needed. I met one of Dr. Feldman's partners, Dr. Read. He was a very articulate man who spoke words five syllables long. But he seemed nice and eager to help.

Then I met Dr. Writer, who was happy to see me. He was the chairman of the hospital credentials committee who had helped me get my application for hospital privileges accepted despite some nasty letters from jealous practitioners in Flatville. He wished me well and, interestingly enough, warned me not to get depressed if there were those around discouraging me. He warned that the community was very political and fighting constantly. I began to think this place was filled with a bunch of savages.

Then there was Dr. Ram, an internist with a special interest in sports medicine. He wanted to be involved with the Bayview Intruders football team and was recommended by Dr. Quackmont. After talking with him I could see he knew nothing about athletic injuries, but I was stuck with him. Dr. Quackmont seemed like he wanted me to use Dr. Ram and I felt I owed Dr. Quackmont this favor. Besides, I needed somebody to help with the day-to-day medical problems for which I had no time, like runny noses and coughs.

Dr. Ram was a complicated man. He was angry and deeply frustrated about something and at times degrading to players. The team administration pressured me on several occasions to either cool him down or to get someone else. Around the hospital he and I were cordial and talked about player problems or upcoming games. He was the only doctor in town that I felt I had some control over. Otherwise, I was clearly the low man on staff. I was ready to head over to my office and begin waiting for the phone to ring when Dr. Quackmont walked into the coffee room. He told me he was happy I had finally arrived and he offered to let me work one to two half-days in the sports medicine clinic where he was the director. I was happy to oblige. I told him I could start immediately.

I mentioned the comment Dr. Small had made that morning and he reassured me that it meant nothing. He also said Dr. Small was never very cordial to competitors. I asked Dr. Quackmont if I could stop by the university to inquire about my application at the student health center, but he said Dr. Small was in charge of the orthopedic situation. He suggested I would be better off talking to Dr. Small directly, even though I had done this previously in his office. I decided to send the application and keep a copy.

I thanked Dr. Quackmont once again for his encouragement in bringing me to Bayview and I told him I was looking forward to seeing him frequently. He expressed an interest in assisting me in surgery, as he prided himself in being a good orthopedic assistant even though he was a family doctor by training. Dr. Laddie walked in as I was ready to leave. He hung his coat on the rack. It looked like he was preparing to stay awhile. He told me about the two patients he had in the hospital and I told him that that was two more than I had. Dr. Quackmont laughed as I got up to leave. "I think you two are going to complement each other nicely," he said.

I spent a few minutes talking to Dr. Laddie and I told him about

Dr. Small's comment. He wasn't surprised. "You didn't think he would welcome you with open arms, did you?" he asked. I asked him if he was going over to the office and he said something I will never forget. "I don't rush over until about 9:45 or 10:00 a.m. That way the 9:00 a.m. patients think I'm busy because they have to wait. Remember, no one likes to see a doctor that isn't busy or they'll think he's no good."

I headed over to the office and ran into Dr. Donner, a local pediatrician in our building. I introduced myself and we chatted for a few minutes. I could tell he had a message for me, even at this early stage. He said he had heard I was coming and that he saw a lot of young people with sports injuries. He promised to send me patients if I was available, but he warned me that Dr. Laddie had no interest in treating kids whatsoever. He said Dr. Laddie told him kids were too noisy and their parents were a bother. Both seemed true enough to me, but I didn't think this was the right time to say so.

He continued, "The entire office found Dr. Laddie very unavailable and parents often had to wait two to three hours for him to respond to a mere phone call. So if you know anything about pediatric orthopedics and you are available, we will make you very busy in a hurry. But I think you'll find out shortly that you need an associate who has the same interest in children's orthopedics as you do. If Dr. Laddie is covering for you, we'll call Dr. Small's group."

On the way upstairs, I pondered my first hour in Bayview. I had been told I wasn't wanted in the community, how hard it was for a young Jewish boy to get started in this anti-Semitic environment, and that it would be wise for me to get a new associate if I wanted to get any business from pediatricians. Maybe I had put on the wrong tie this morning.

Well, already I was not following the advice of Dr. Feldman. It was 9:15 a.m. and I was late getting to the office. I was ready for my first day in private practice. But I had no patients. My secretary welcomed me and said she was excited. I had given her a new lease on life. She was happy to be away from Dr. Ley and I was happy to have her. She knew about medical offices and how to bill medical insurances. I felt confident in her abilities. I was asking her to do a lot, though, scheduling the patients, answering the phone, and billing the insurance companies. Luckily, I wasn't too busy or she might quit.

Fortunately for me, things started to happen fast. I could never do well sitting around waiting for the phone to ring. We had a few aces in the hole. My secretary's husband came through, as he called within ten minutes to ask if I could see a football player with a sprained knee. Absolutely. I hadn't even met her husband, Gervin, but he sure sounded like a nice, positive fellow. I suggested we have lunch that week.

I also got a call from Dr. Read, who had just admitted a lady to the hospital with terrible back pain and wondered if I was too busy to see this consult. Not at all.

I was off and running. Between my Gervin connection, doctors feeling sorry for me, and meeting several referring doctors each day, I was doing well within a month. The phone began to ring constantly. Also, I had let it be known that I was more than happy to be an assistant in surgery, day or night. The neurosurgeons frequently called me to assist on back operations. These were great because they paid well.

It became obvious to me that I would not be able to continue doing this type of assisting very long. If I was in surgery and assisting other doctors, I wasn't available to see patients on a moment's notice for people like Dr. Feldman. He saw me one day and said he had tried to send me a patient, but I was helping in surgery so he had had to send the patient to one of my competitors. This was said to make me feel bad and to send a message that I better listen to the advice he gave me if I wanted to succeed in this town. Little did I know that he would be the first in a line of many who would disagree with my priorities in medicine.

I decided I should be in practice for a few months and keep my nose to the grindstone without rocking the boat. Essentially, this meant doing everything the way other docs wanted me to do them and not concerning myself with what I thought was proper or right. But as time went on, this became increasingly hard, and before long I began to exert my priorities forcefully.

Dr. Laddie had hired a young x-ray technician long before I arrived. I hadn't been in practice two months when she approached me at lunch one day while Dr. Laddie was away. "You know, Dr. Mays, Dr. Laddie promised me a big raise before you came and he has never lived up to his promise. I think you'll agree I'm a very good x-ray technician. I do a lot of extra typing and I'm deserving of a big raise," she concluded. I had never liked this little bitch from the day I'd started. She was snippy and short with patients, frequently late in the morning, and dashed out the door promptly at 5:00 p.m. She got along poorly with the other employees in the office. I knew what I had to do. This would be my first major office decision. She would be gone in two weeks. But for the time being, I said, "I'll discuss this with Dr. Laddie and see exactly what he promised you."

I could afford to be a little cocky. I had treated a patient, Sue Ellen, a few days ago who was an x-ray technician in a nearby town. I was excited about this lady. She was a runner with shin splints, a weight lifter, single, and she lived two blocks from the office. I asked her how she liked working at her present job. She said that most of the patients were indigent and she had been looking to change jobs, so I asked if I could call her should a job become available. She seemed interested.

It all happened quickly. Although my mind was made up, I spoke with Dr. Laddie just to get his feedback. He stated that he had never promised her a raise and he too was less than impressed with her performance and attitude. So we hired Sue Ellen and gave our snippy x-ray technician the boot.

This was the first major principle I learned in private practice. The best resource for good employees is your patients. Sue Ellen arrived at work on time and was pleasant to the patients. I trained her to do other tasks in the office such as changing dressings and helping to put on casts. She typed our chart dictations when she was not taking x-rays and kept track of all the supplies in the office. Most importantly, she took better x-rays than our previous technician.

Tension continued to mount between Dr. Small's group and myself. They wanted to be rid of me, frequently making derogatory statements to doctors who referred patients to me in an attempt to destroy my reputation. "Dr. Mays is too aggressive with the knife. Don't send your patients to him or he'll operate on them," they continually advised.

I was becoming the major recipient of orthopedic referrals and I had clearly taken over the majority of arthroscopic work from Dr. Stalin. Also, I continued to get major publicity as the team physician for the Intruders. I was a big thorn in the side of Dr. Small and his gang.

Every Monday morning, Dr. Small would meet with his troops

in a secluded corner in the hospital to talk about office matters. But I knew much of the discussion was centered on me and how best to destroy my practice. I became very busy in short order. I had pulled out all the stops and made it happen. I focused in on one concept: the patient is number one. I remember the day I saw a new patient in my office and I asked her how she was referred to me. She said I had operated on the foot of a lady who worked in her office. She had never forgotten how this lady returned to work the day after surgery and told everyone her doctor had called her at home the night of surgery just to see how she was doing. Everyone in the office was so impressed. She assured me I would be seeing other members of her office in the future. Mission accomplished.

As was the case with all new physicians on the hospital staff, I had to be proctored on my first six surgical cases. This meant that another orthopedist, and not Dr. Laddie, had to watch me operate to make sure I didn't mutilate a patient. You can imagine what a thrill it was to call one of my competitors to proctor me while I pinned a hip on a patient referred by a doctor who used to refer to them.

Dr. Small's group didn't want to go out of their way to help me, but I was busy enough that I finished my proctoring within a month. Of course no one reported that I was an excellent surgeon or that I had incredible skills, but rather that the surgery had been performed adequately and I had had no complications.

I would stop by the emergency room as much as possible, but I had to pick my times carefully so I wouldn't run into Dr. Ley's mistress, Cobra. By now she had spread her venom throughout the entire department, saying that I was an incompetent orthopedist who was causing big trouble in the community. But what could I expect? I let it be known that I was aware of the inappropriate referrals Dr. Ley was receiving and, in fact, the administration had received the evidence that Nordy had accumulated. Once the situation was reviewed, Cobra was severely reprimanded for her unethical behavior and was moved out of the emergency department to the outpatient surgery clinic. Needless to say, in over five years, this lady has not said one word to me.

My practice was growing by leaps and bounds, and I learned a very important lesson in practice. Never let the opposition know how you are doing. I accomplished this by not commenting on my busy practice and by using different hospitals so that the doctors in surgery, like the anesthesiologist, weren't able to tell I was busy. I took one case to Bayview and the next case across town, etc.

Between the Bayview Intruders and Gervin's college football team, life was becoming as busy as I had hoped. I was seeing a lot of athletic injuries from the college and I couldn't have asked for a greater group of kids. Many of the students had surgical injuries and most of them could be fixed with a good result. This served as a great advertisement in itself.

I got a kick out of these "underprivileged" students. This college was a rich kids' institution. Many of my patients drove to my office in Porsches and Mercedes. They paid with credit cards from mommy and daddy, and the classes they took impressed me no end. One young, pretty co-ed had a rough semester because she had two physical education classes, first aid, California literature, and philosophy.

Our office was crowded, mainly because we only had two exam rooms, and Dr. Laddie and I had very different styles. I spent ten to fifteen minutes with each patient and moved along quickly. He sat down in the exam room, propped his feet up on the stool, and chatted with patients for as long as forty-five minutes. This was a problem when I was trying to move patients in and out of the office.

We also had a satellite office in Casa, where I began to spend more time. I wasn't as busy there but I was interested in expanding my operation, and it was closer to the college where Gervin worked. It also made sense to spend afternoons in this community because most athletic activities at the college, like intramural sports and team practices, took place in the afternoons. I wanted to be available for these injured warriors. Gervin was so busy in the training room that an athlete with any sort of pain was sent to me for evaluation.

There was no question that the greatest thing about Nordy was her husband. She was a good secretary and helped me get started, but many of the patients thought she was loud and rude on the telephone and my accountant was less than impressed with her record-keeping abilities. He spent more time correcting her mistakes than he did figuring out my taxes and expenses.

There was one patient Gervin sent who would change my life. Bud, a varsity basketball player, had dislocated his shoulder on numerous occasions and had previously been sent to another orthopedist before I came to town. He came to me for a second opinion, although he had already set up a surgery date with the other doctor. Bud was pleasant and had a legitimate problem that needed surgery, but I was most impressed with his father, Mr. Bright. This gentleman had traveled over one hundred miles to hear the second surgical opinion about his son. It was obvious that he took a genuine interest in his boy and I was deeply touched by his soft-spoken nature and sensitive involvement. Their closeness was demonstrated by their interaction as we discussed the pros and cons of surgical intervention, the possible complications, and, of course, Bud's chances for returning to basketball. Before they left I was informed that they wanted me to do the surgery immediately. I didn't think much about it and off they went.

The following week, I performed the shoulder reconstruction on Bud and fortunately all went well. As I was writing postoperative orders in the chart, I noticed on the face sheet, written under the heading "Occupation," Discovery Point Golf Club. This was one of the most prestigious and famous golf courses in the entire world. I wondered if Bud had a part-time job there in the summer. I was envious, as I had always wanted to set foot on this very private course. I finished the orders and set out to find his dad. I found him in the surgery waiting room with his wife. I told them things had gone well and, hopefully, in about three months Bud would be able to return to collegiate basketball. They seemed ecstatic and I told them I would stop by to check on Bud before I went home.

As I departed, I asked, "By the way, what does Bud do at Discovery Point Golf Club?" Mr. Bright laughed and said, "Oh, that's where I work. I'm the golf professional there." I had just operated on the son of the golf professional at Discovery Point. If his kid had any complication from surgery, I was going to kill myself. I had a legitimate chance of landing a starting time at Discovery Point, the place most golfers only dreamed about playing. I was stoked.

Over the next several months, I struck up a close relationship with the Brights. Believe it or not, this had very little to do with the golf course. These people were so unique and caring that it was difficult not to treat them in a special way. Mr. Bright frequently drove up to watch the basketball games with Bud while he was recuperating and I was invited to the games with them.

And then, unexpectedly, Mr. Bright asked if I would ever consider driving down to play Discovery Point. At first, I laughed. Typical Mr. Bright, he always made the other person feel good. He continued, "I would be so honored to have you and three friends come down to play sometime soon. After all, everyone at the club has heard so much about you that I want them all to meet you." I couldn't figure out how to say to this man that he had just made my day. I told him I was so excited I wouldn't be able to sleep for a week, and that I would cancel an appointment with the president of the United States to play golf at Discovery Point.

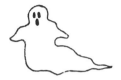

24. Ghost Surgery

MY RELATIONSHIP with Dr. Laddie started off well. I knew very little about him except that his practice was slow and he lived and breathed golf. He was pleasant to talk with and never in a hurry. I could see he would be no competition.

His office secretaries were an unusual bunch. Dot, his first secretary, was bossy and drove Nordy crazy. When Dot's health started to deteriorate, she retired. She was replaced by Bea, a black lady who was very quiet but loyal. But when Dr. Laddie took the big plunge and decided to get a computer, the salesman/owner of the company, Mr. Club, made some prejudicial remarks to Bea and she quit.

The joke was on Dr. Laddie, because the computer ended up costing him over $100,000. Mr. Club sold Dr. Laddie a lemon and the computer couldn't send out bills for over a year. Dr. Laddie's patients loved this as they would see him several times a year for free. Most patients had huge deductibles on their insurance plans and his computer wasn't keeping track.

Dr. Laddie finally settled on another computer and a new office manager, Iata. She was a certified travel agent and was specifically looking for a job where the doctor wasn't busy and was frequently gone so she could conduct her travel business on the side. With his declining patient load and the computer functioning, she could take care of her travel clients. She got along well with my office staff.

His secretaries had one major instruction when it came to booking surgeries. They had to make sure that I was available to help. Nordy was the first to alert me to this as she would frequently ask about moving my patients around to accommodate Dr. Laddie's surgery schedule. I had only been in Bayview a few months when the reason for this became clear.

Dr. Laddie and I were performing a total hip replacement on one of his patients when, shortly after the case started, he asked me to ream out the hip socket. "It's much easier to ream from your side of the operating table," he said. Not thinking much of it, I obliged since I was a lot younger than he and this took some strength. But later in the case, he asked me to ream the thigh bone before the insertion of the final metallic prosthesis and this was clearly easier from his side. I did it again because he had recently been diagnosed with a serious illness and I thought maybe he wasn't feeling well. But I became troubled as this happened more and more. These were his patients and I was doing more of the surgery than he.

This became increasingly obvious, especially with arthroscopic surgery. I was clearly the "guru" in Bayview when it came to arthroscopy and my average case took less than twenty minutes. Dr. Laddie trained long before arthroscopy was invented, so he learned arthroscopy by watching video tapes. His cases took one to two hours and he was very clumsy with the instruments. He would frequently say, "It'll take me a half hour to cut out this torn cartilage when you can do it in five minutes. Why don't you just go ahead and finish this so we can get out of here?" So I would.

This went on for five years. My reasons for doing it were numerous. I felt sorry that Dr. Laddie had already missed several months of practice while he was undergoing medical treatment. I knew he needed the money badly as he frequently mentioned how he would soon need a loan at this pace. Second, he was not a technically superior orthopedic surgeon. And finally, time was a terrible problem because Dr. Laddie operated so slowly. Even tying knots was an adventure for him. So if I didn't want to spend the rest of the day standing at the operating table, I would do the case just to get done. I simply didn't know how to say no. I frequently wondered how to get out of this situation. I asked the advice of several close doctor friends and their responses were unanimous. It was wrong and needed to stop immediately. Many said that I had allowed it to go on too long and there was constant talk around the hospital and Surgicenter that I was doing all of Dr. Laddie's work.

I decided to take the plunge one Friday afternoon when we were both finished with patients and all of the secretaries had gone home. The atmosphere was friendly, so I asked Dr. Laddie if he had a few minutes to chat. I told him how difficult it was to bring up this subject, but I was extremely uncomfortable doing surgery on his patients. I stated it was dishonest to tell patients he would be doing the surgery and it put the facility in an unfair position from a medical-legal standpoint. I mentioned that from a financial point of view, it was a losing proposition for me, since I was only able to bill for the assistant surgeon's fee and he received five times that as the surgeon. Even worse, the assistant surgeon's fee for an arthroscopy was often denied by insurance companies. There were many instances when I did the case for free.

I was dumbfounded when Dr. Laddie said, "I really don't understand what you mean, Buck. I know that occasionally you do small parts of the case, but I do virtually all my own surgery." I could see he was angry.

So I took another approach and said, "In any event, I can't continue to assist you at surgery unless you agree to a system that's fair to both of us. If you're uncomfortable with a specific surgical procedure like arthroscopy, tell the patient your associate does a lot of it and refer the patient to me. I'll bill for the surgery, you bill the assistant's fee and we'll split the total purse fifty-fifty." This seemed fair to me. He said he wasn't interested and thought my idea was childish. He added that he might not be as fast as me at arthroscopy, but he was definitely as good, and if that was the way I felt about our relationship, he didn't need my help anymore. He grabbed his coat and walked out.

I was stunned, initially, but knew it was for the best. I felt better about myself and I knew my liability had decreased significantly. I was unsure of the impact it would have on Dr. Laddie's practice. For a period of four months, he did no arthroscopies.

Six months after our meeting, I was traveling with the football team when a patient of mine injured his left knee. I had previously done arthroscopy on his right knee. Dr. Laddie saw him in the office on Saturday with a locked knee and suggested it would be best to look in the knee on Monday with the arthroscope. My patient wanted to wait for my return, but Dr. Laddie told him and his mother I would not be back until Tuesday. The patient reluctantly consented to Dr. Laddie operating on Monday.

When I returned Tuesday morning, my answering service told me I was to immediately contact the medical director at the Surgicenter. I called Dr. Snootful and he was angry. He told me Dr. Laddie had no business doing arthroscopy alone and that when he had called to schedule the case, the Surgicenter had assumed that I would be in attendance. It wasn't until he was thirty minutes into the case that the nurse asked when I would be there. Dr. Laddie said I was out of town.

Dr. Laddie finished the case in just over three hours. The patient stayed in the recovery room another two hours with significant pain. Dr. Snootful said that the mother was livid and suggested I call her immediately. I did so and she was outraged that Dr. Laddie had insisted the surgery be done immediately to prevent significant harm to her son's knee. I told her I was very sorry that I hadn't been available when they needed me, and as soon as I had a chance to speak with Dr. Laddie, I would call her back.

I waited for him to wander over from the coffee room; he finally arrived about 10:00 a.m. He made no mention of the case and barely said hello. After twenty minutes, I finally asked him. He said, "Oh yes, I almost forgot. Your patient came in on Saturday with a locked knee and I told him he could wait for you on Tuesday or I could take a look at it on Monday. They didn't want to wait so I scoped him yesterday. He had a bucket handle tear of his cartilage that was stuck in the back of the knee. I think even you would have had trouble with this one. It took me a little longer than usual, but he'll do just fine." He walked out of the room.

My secretary said the head nurse was on the phone from the Surgicenter. She asked me if I had heard about Dr. Laddie's case and I conveyed what I had heard from Dr. Laddie, the mother, and Dr. Snootful. She said it was horrible. The staff was terrified because Dr. Laddie could not get the job done and was cursing and sweating and no one knew what to do. Then she said something that really jolted me. She admitted she was no expert in arthroscopy, but she doubted the cartilage was fixed from what she saw on the video screen during surgery.

I called the mother back and asked her to bring her son to the office that afternoon so I could see the knee and we could all talk. I spent over an hour with them and calmed them as best I could. But I was disturbed over the appearance of the knee. It was warm and swollen. Most arthroscopic patients walked into the office the day following surgery without crutches. This patient could bear no weight on the operated leg.

I saw him again one week later and he was worse. Something had to be wrong. Here was a very athletic boy who couldn't even hobble on his leg. He was dejected and his mother was mad. I told them this was a difficult situation and that it would be best for me to operate again and identify the problem. I assured them there would be no charge. I said nothing negative about Dr. Laddie but continued to wonder why he had insisted on doing this case. They reluctantly agreed and we scheduled surgery for the next day. As suspected, he had a severely displaced tear in the cartilage which hadn't been fixed. I repaired the problem in fifteen minutes and he left an hour later, partially bearing weight without crutches. I assured the mother he would make a quick recovery.

One week later, he came back to have his stitches removed. He walked back to physical therapy in our office without a limp. The mother stayed behind and asked if she could have a word with me. We sat down in my consultation room and shut the door. She thanked me profusely for taking care of this problem and informed me that she was filing a lawsuit against Dr. Laddie.

I told her I understood her position but asked if she would hear me out. I explained that Dr. Laddie hadn't been feeling well and he shouldn't have performed this operation. She asked how the next innocent patient would be spared. I told her the problem had been addressed at the Surgicenter and if she wanted confirmation of that she could call Dr. Snootful. I pleaded that it would be a personal favor to me to forget this whole experience and to drop the lawsuit. She said that because of my concern and the care I had given them over the years that she would back off.

I saw Dr. Laddie in the coffee room the following day. Somehow he had heard about our mutual patient having a second surgery. He asked what I found in the knee. I said that another piece of cartilage must have broken loose after the surgery, so I went back in and took care of it. He said he was surprised since everything had looked great when he left. He hoped the family wasn't too discouraged with another surgery.

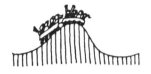

25. Rollercoaster

So, you want to be a doctor? What is my typical day like?

4:35 a.m. Is this a dream? What's ringing? Oh, Christ, it's the telephone. "Hello, Dr. Mays, it's your answering service. Your patient, Mr. Miller, is on the line. He says the cast you put on today is too tight." Okay. I guess I have to take the call.

"Hello, Dr. Mays, is that you?" Mr. Miller asks. (No, it's the colonel from Kentucky Fried Chicken.) "Yes," I scream with my eyes shut. "My cast is still as tight as it was when you put it on this afternoon. Since I couldn't sleep, I thought I should call you, because I have to go to work in the morning," he continues. And I don't? "Are you keeping the arm elevated?" I ask. "Well, I did this afternoon, but my shoulder hurts from holding it up, so I've held it down for the past several hours," he says. I suggest that this non-compliant patient put the arm up on several pillows and keep it elevated like I told him. If it is still too tight, I'll split it—either the cast or his head!

6:15 a.m. My alarm goes off. Is it time to get up, already? I seem to recall the telephone ringing a few hours ago, but I can't for the life of me remember what it was all about. A regular necktie will have to do today, because with all that surgery, I don't want to have to tie my bow tie over and over again. It takes too long. No sweater vest either. Dressing takes too long.

7:00 a.m. Making rounds at the hospital is exciting. "Does anyone know what Mrs. Munoz's temperature is?" I ask the ward nurse. I'm told I can't find out the temperature right now because all of the nurses are in report. When I enter the nurses' room, you should see the looks I get. When I ask about the temperature, one of the nurses replies, "We were so short-staffed last night, Dr. Mays, that we had all we could do to pass out the medications. We didn't take any temperatures. Sorry." I'm wondering if anyone even saw Mrs. Munoz last night or if she's still alive. Well, since all else has failed, I guess I'd better go look at the patient myself. Fortunately, she looks good.

I'll go see if Mr. Bright's toes are warm after that commando operation to plate the unhealed bone in his leg. The beeper goes off on the way to his room. It's the emergency room telling me I have a referral, an eighty-five-year-old lady with a fractured hip. "I'll be down in a few minutes." I see my day becoming chaotic already.

I ask the nurse in Mr. Bright's room why the incentive spirometer that I ordered postoperatively to help expand his lungs is not at his bedside. "That was supposed to be delivered by the respiratory therapist, Dr. Mays, and they didn't make it by last night," she says. Hey, no big deal. So the patient gets an embolism to his lungs or his brain after surgery and dies. Or he has to be in the intensive care unit for a week on blood thinners, if he survives.

7:20 a.m. I rush to the emergency room before heading to the Surgicenter for my 7:30 a.m. case. "Hello, Mrs. Jamison. I'm Dr. Mays. I'm a bone doctor. You've broken your hip and we need to fix it so you can walk again," I explain to this elderly lady lying on the gurney. Her daughter is looking at me strangely. "Excuse me Doctor, but you look so young. How many of these hip operations have you done?" she asks. "Thank you for saying I look so young, but let me assure you I have had a great deal of experience since graduating from the university, where I did over 150 of these hip pinnings," I reassure her. The poor lady fell this morning on the way to the kitchen and has not had anything to eat or drink. I'll add her name to the surgery schedule and fix it around five o'clock tonight. Fat chance. Not the way the surgery department at Bayview General is run.

7:25 a.m. As I pick up the phone in the emergency room, I realize I'm supposed to be operating in five minutes at the Surgicenter a few miles away. I'll jump in the car and dictate an admission note and schedule the surgery on this lady from my car phone. Not a cheap toy, but it saves me time. "Good morning. This is Dr. Mays. I'd like to schedule a five o'clock hip pinning," I explain to the scheduling nurse. I'm told they have overscheduled in surgery today and the surgeon doing the last case is notoriously slow.

7:31 a.m. I can't believe it. This light in front of the doughnut shop is always red and I've never seen a soul coming in the other direction.

7:34 a.m. "Good morning," I say as I rush into surgery. The patient is already asleep. He's a young football player with recurrent snapping in his left knee and a positive magnetic resonance test for a torn cartilage.

7:39 a.m. The arthroscopy begins after I scrub my hands. The camera, television, and all the tools work. The Surgicenter is great. Anything outside Bayview Hospital seems to work better. Here we have fewer postoperative complications, less resistance from the staff, and a more pleasant environment. The tear in the medial meniscus is obvious, so we will just switch to the end cutter and cut it away.

7:48 a.m. "Okay, lights on. Let's close," I tell the scrub nurse. That worked out well. I'll have time for a cup of coffee and then back to the hospital for more rounds.

Can you believe it! The damn beeper is going off again. It's the orthopedic nurse at Bayview General. I forgot to order bowel care for one of my patients. "Mrs. Reddin can have bowel care of choice," I say. That nurse is like a drill sergeant. I wish for just a day I could order routine bowel care for her. Nothing fancy. Just an enema every two minutes over the next four days, whether she needs it or not.

8:15 a.m. I'll stop in the coffee room for a minute before I go sign my charts. I seem to be getting the cold shoulder from the in-house doctors, like the radiologist, cardiologist, and anesthesiologist. They're upset because I participated in the opening of a new off-site x-ray unit that competes with the hospital and reduces their ability to make money. "Good morning Tim," I say. He doesn't answer me. He's sitting down at the other end of the table hiding his face behind the financial section of the paper. He's an in-house doctor who stands to lose thousands of dollars a year if I send all my x-ray studies away from the hospital. But that will give him more time to study the stock market. I understand he suffered big losses on some previous investments.

8:25 a.m. At the medical records room, I don't see the charts I ordered last Friday. "Do you know if anyone has pulled my charts?" I inquire. The girl at the desk asks my name. After all, I've only been on staff at this hospital for five years. Why should I expect anybody to know my name? She explains that the girl who worked on Friday and who normally pulls all of the charts is sick today so no one knows whether or not my charts were pulled. She looks in the file. "You have six charts," she notes. "Please sit down and I'll get them for you right away."

I see one of the chest doctors signing charts over in the corner. I'll walk over and say hello. He begins telling me how inappropriate my orders are on patients following major surgery. He says I don't need to order both respiratory therapy treatments and a spirometer for the patient. "But why not?" I ask. He explains that if they can do one, they don't need the other. I angrily respond, "You must realize that many orthopedic patients are elderly and incoherent right after surgery. If the therapist doesn't come by to assist them, they won't deep-breathe and cough at all. They never remember to use the spirometer unless the nurse is standing right in front of them. By ordering both the chance of some deep breathing and coughing taking place is fifty percent more likely." He shakes his head at me. Of course I'll continue to order both whether he likes it or not.

8:31 a.m. Oh, good. Here comes the medical records lady. "Hi, Dr. Mays," she says. "I have no charts for you. I can't locate two of your charts and one is in the cardiologist's office for dictation. One is pulled for another doctor who was supposed to dictate on it last week, and two are out to the utilization review committee for insurance purposes. So none of your charts are available for signature, Dr. Mays. Can I be of any further assistance to you?" she smiles.

8:34 a.m. I need another cup of coffee. The same complainers are in the coffee room telling us how medicine has changed and how hard it is to earn a living. Let's see. The guy in the brown sports jacket drives a Porsche. The pathologist in the green dress drives a Mercedes station wagon, and the surgeon eating the doughnut has a BMW convertible. It seems the biggest complainers have the biggest, most expensive cars.

8:55 a.m. I love my secretaries. Look, it's ten minutes before nine and they're already here. "Do you want an x-ray on Mrs. Hart, Dr. Mays? She's the lady who fell off the horse last week," my technician asks. That seems like a good idea since the fracture is only five days old and we need to check the alignment of the bones.

"Eugene, what are you doing without your brace on?" I scold. He's got the typical high school football player mentality. Three weeks following a complicated knee ligament reconstruction, he leaves his brace off and is walking with all his weight on the operated leg. He's not supposed to be walking on it for eight weeks. He doesn't even bring the brace to the office. "It feels great, Doc. I've even started a little jogging with the football team," he brags.

His mother is on the phone. She tells me Eugene will not cooperate with the postoperative instructions. She asks that I be very firm with him and adds that if this operation fails because of his lack of cooperation, she won't be able to afford another one. "He can pay for it himself, or let his father pay," she says. I scold Eugene about his brace and warn him never to come back to my office without it on for the next eight weeks.

9:20 a.m. Harry is here for another social call. He broke his wrist about six months ago, but he wants me to check it again. It looks as good as it did three months ago. But someday I will be old and wish someone would listen to me. I like my older patients. They are charming and they don't ask a lot of unreasonable questions. I reassure Harry that everything is okay and to please drop by around the holidays.

9:25 a.m. Well, let's see a new patient. "Hi, Doctor. My knee was bothering me about three months ago when I made this appointment, but it feels fine now. Since I had the appointment scheduled, I wanted to ask you about my lower back, which has been bothering me for the past ten years. And my husband thinks my bunions are getting worse and they should be fixed, even though they don't hurt me," she states. I immediately think of a suggestion. Tie your two big toes together, which will arch your back, which will abduct your thighs, so your husband can take his frigging eyes off your bunions!

10:15 a.m. I get a call from Dr. Feldman. He wants to send down one of his private patients who is a Nobel laureate with a lump on his wrist. The patient thinks he has cancer. "Send him down," I suggest. I never turn down a new patient with insurance.

My secretary tells me that there is a patient on the telephone who is annoyed with me for prescribing a medicine that made his stomach upset. He admits, however, that he forgot to take the pills with meals. "Let's try another medication, and this time try to remember to take it with food," I suggest. I told him this the last time he was in the office, but he was too busy asking questions to listen.

10:45 a.m. I'm explaining to this lady whose shoulder keeps

dislocating that she needs an operation. It has come out of the socket six times, the last one while she was reaching for a can of Coke in the refrigerator. "My brother, who is a laboratory technician in Boston, says I probably have tendinitis and you should be giving me medication," she says. Okay. The customer is always right. I'll send you to physical therapy and put you on some medication. You can pay me now or pay me later.

11:05 a.m. "Good morning. I'm Dr. Mays," I greet an elderly lady. She explains that she has been unable to move her shoulder for the past several months and she's had no injury. Her exam shows the typical signs of bursitis with decreased range of motion, stiffness, and pain. Since she has been taking enough aspirin to give her ulcers, I explain the best treatment would be a cortisone shot. "My son, who is an attorney, said that whatever I do, don't get a cortisone shot because they hurt like hell and the doctor uses a needle about a foot long," she states. Of course everything is a foot long to an attorney until he stands in front of a mirror nude. Then he learns to measure things in millimeters.

I assure her that the shot wouldn't hurt and if it does, there would be no charge. Occasionally, I'm wrong, but what the hell if the patient can't take a joke. "Well, I can't brush my teeth or fasten my bra with this arm, so go ahead," she says. She leaves the office in no pain with the shoulder moving almost normally and realizing her son's a big wimp.

11:15 a.m. "There's a call from that attorney again about your court appearance as an expert witness," my secretary says. My policy about depositions and court appearances is clear. All fees are paid up front. Why? Because most of these cases settle out of court at the last minute and I'm sitting there holding the proverbial bag with no patients scheduled and no money. By collecting up front, my nonrefundable fee covers my empty calendar.

11:20 a.m. "I'll bet you're tired of this cast, Jamie," I say as she giggles. She broke her wrist falling off a skateboard four weeks ago and is back to have her cast removed. I explain to her that the cast saw makes a lot of noise, but it won't cut her, and I show her on my own skin first. I reassure her that the wrist will do fine, but to take it easy over the next few weeks while the muscles get stronger. I suggest that she refrain from contact sports like football, soccer, and dating over the next two weeks. Oh yes, she needs another excuse for P.E., because now that the cast is off, her teacher won't believe she had a broken wrist.

11:25 a.m. I'll check out the high school kid who injured his wrist and nose yesterday in a football game. The doctor on the sideline pushed the nose back straight and told the kid he was fine. Get back into the game. Let's x-ray the wrist. It's cracked and I suggest that for quickest healing, he be in a cast for four weeks and not play. His mother is a nurse and his father is a physician. They agree. Unfortunately, this young man is the star player on the team, so he bullies his parents into letting him play without the cast. I'm in disbelief, but it's not my wrist. I have to laugh because these parents frequently boast how level-headed their children are. And I'm a captain for United Airlines.

11:30 a.m. "Well, what happened to you?" I ask. Mr. Dumars explains that his wife made him so mad that he hit the wall, instead of her. That is one swollen hand if I ever saw one. I can't believe an accountant could be so violent. "Don't you folks just play with numbers, tell us how poorly we're doing financially, and say that the tax situation has worsened over the past year?" I joke. On examination, the little finger is pointing toward the thumb, which I recall is not anatomically correct. "Let's get an x-ray," I say. It shows a severe, unstable, spiral fracture of the finger that will require open reduction and internal fixation with two or three pins. He wants to do it today. I'll call the Surgicenter and see if I can add him on at noon and do it under local anesthesia. They have one local room available. So much for lunch.

11:45 a.m. Between patients, I open the mail and return phone calls. The lady whose bunion I operated on three days ago is calling to ask about the pin which is holding her bone straight. "How far out the end of my toe should the pin be sticking?" she asks. "Just far enough to improve your television reception, sweetheart," I quip. "How are you going to pull this pin out? Will it hurt?" she asks. "It won't hurt me a bit," I laugh.

The nurses in surgery at Bayview want to know what instruments I will be needing for the total knee replacement next week. "Don't you gals have my case cards there? I have been doing these for the past five years," I complain. They explain that all of my cards have been lost or misplaced. I immediately wonder if my competitors had anything to do with that. This would never happen at the Surgicenter.

11:55 a.m. I'd better get over to the Surgicenter and fix the finger. As I get out of the car, I realize I forgot the x-rays and turn around to go back. My wonderful secretary meets me in the parking lot with the films and wishes me good luck. I have the best team in town.

On the way back to the Surgicenter, I decide to call and see if my patient ever had her temperature taken. "Hi, Dr. Mays, please hold the line," the ward clerk answers. I hate when I have to hold on the car phone. It's expensive. It's cheaper to hang up and call back, so I do. "Four Northwest, please hold," the ward clerk answers again. She finally comes back in four minutes (and $4 later) to tell me that she looked all over for my patient's nurse and then realized she was at lunch.

I'm wondering if it ever dawned on this stupid woman to look at the chart. "I wonder if you could just look at the patient's chart and see if her temperature has been taken," I ask. "That's a good idea, Dr. Mays," she says. I want to throw the car phone through the window. I decide I don't want to know the temperature that badly and hang up the phone.

12:03 p.m. "Hi, Doc, they are ready for you in room one," the head nurse at the Surgicenter states. We fix the finger in twenty minutes, and after dictating the operative report, I find a sandwich waiting for me in the surgeons' lounge. If the hospital ever bought me a sandwich, I would probably pass out.

As I begin to take a bite, my beeper goes off. It's one of the family doctors calling to say that he has a very disoriented seventy-five-year-old lady, Mrs. Glover, whose daughter noticed she was limping. He sent them to the outpatient radiology department at the hospital and the radiologist said the hip is broken. "I sent her to admitting. Could you see her for me?" he asks.

I agree and tell him I will call over to the hospital and make sure this lady is NPO (does not eat). I'll order two units of blood for hip surgery and add her onto the schedule to follow the other fractured hip I'm doing this evening. I'd better change my clothes and get to the hospital. I can eat my sandwich in the car.

12:35 p.m. I decide to call admitting at the hospital and see if this lady arrived yet. "Dr. Mays, do you really think this patient needs to come to the hospital now? We have a shortage of beds and she has been walking around on the broken hip anyway," the admissions clerk asks. I beg for a room on the orthopedic floor, but they give her the only available bed in the entire hospital. It's in the respiratory intensive care unit.

12:55 p.m. I can't find the lady with the broken hip. She's not in the waiting room, the emergency room, admitting, or in the lab. "Which room was Mrs. Glover assigned?" I ask the admissions secretary. "She hasn't arrived yet, Dr. Mays, but we have been notified by her family doctor that she is supposed to arrive any minute," she says. Great, I'll grab a cup of coffee in the doctors' lunchroom before my afternoon patients.

1:10 p.m. I'll check once more at the admitting office and see whatever happened to Mrs. Glover. Admitting says that she just checked in and is waiting for the transportation person to take her upstairs to the ward. I'm told that she's a pleasant lady wearing a bright orange sweater and sitting in a blue wheelchair. But where is she? How far could she have gone?

1:15 p.m. How long have I been looking for this lady? How could these idiots waste my time like this? Screw it. I'll go look at her x-rays and to hell with the patient. When I arrive in x-ray, I'm told by the technician that the patient has the films and she's riding around in a blue wheelchair.

I'll head back over to my office. As I'm strolling down the hallway, I can't believe what I see. In the cafeteria, there is a lady wearing a bright orange sweater, sitting in a blue wheelchair, eating a full plate of spaghetti. "Excuse me, but you wouldn't happen to be Mrs. Glover, by chance?" I ask. "Yes sir, she is, and I'm her daughter," her companion answers. "What are you doing?" I lecture. "You were not supposed to have any food so I could fix your hip tonight, but it's too late now. The surgery will have to be postponed until tomorrow." So much for patient compliance.

1:20 p.m. Walking back to my office, I ask myself if I'm having fun yet. As I cross the street, a local family doctor appears to ignore me. He's on a health plan committee that gives prior authorization for orthopedic procedures. I publicly objected to this committee, which has two family doctors and a chest surgeon deciding which orthopedic procedures are necessary.

The medical director of the Hopeless Health Plan felt that too much money was being spent on orthopedic procedures, so he persuaded some friends to sit on this committee to slow the process down. He thought that if procedures were questioned long enough, patients might change their minds. Why don't they call me to approve insulin for diabetics or see if the heart surgeons have the proper indications to do their cardiac bypass procedures?

As I walk in the back door of my office, I see three people sitting in the waiting room. I'm already behind schedule.

1:23 p.m. My first patient is a young man who tells me his mother sent him in to ask some questions about his knee. "She wants to know if you think my knee will get better as time goes on," he says. It's probably a stupid question, but I'll ask anyway. "Where's your mother today?" "She's at her tennis lesson. She wanted to come, but this is the only day the club pro teaches," he responds. "Well, how did you get here?" I ask. "I rode the bus. I only had to transfer three times and it took less than two hours to get here." I'm wondering exactly what his mother is doing with the pro and whether he might be stringing her racket a little tighter! I spend over twenty minutes explaining about the instability in his knee from ligament damage. I'm sure he'll tell Mommy, who will then most certainly give me a call to say she is not sure she got the straight facts from her son. I'll have to explain this all over again. Parents like this drive me wild!

1:47 p.m. "What's all the commotion?" I ask while running out of the exam room. My secretaries look hysterical and people are dashing around in the waiting room. "A patient just limped through the front door and is crying in pain, Dr. Mays," one secretary shouts.

It's an elderly gentleman who was out walking on a nearby trail and fell. "I was going to the emergency room, Doc, but figured you could help me more since it's my back that hurts," he says lying on the floor. Smart man. He doesn't want to waste time and he knows if he goes to the emergency room, he'll wait at least three hours to see a doctor, then be sent to x-ray, and he still won't have seen a specialist. He's got the system figured out. If you crawl into a doctor's office, there's a good chance you'll be seen promptly. "Let me help you into the x-ray room and we'll get some pictures," I offer.

We learn that this guy crawled two miles to my office. X-rays show two broken ribs and a fractured vertebra. I admit him to the hospital for overnight observation and pain control. I'm now behind forty-five minutes with my office appointments.

2:30 p.m. A local pediatrician is on the phone. There's a seven-year-old girl in his office who just fell off the monkey bars at school and her wrist is crooked. "I'd like to send her over right away," he says.

2:35 p.m. My next patient is a young man who just twisted his ankle playing basketball. "What's going on, big guy?" I ask. His father interrupts by saying he has done this many times before. "Show me where it hurts," I interrupt his father. The father shows me where the black-and-blue marks are on the ankle. Isn't it aggravating? Parents don't think their kids can speak for themselves. "I wonder if I could talk with Dan for a minute?" I ask. Dad gives me a dirty look. After speaking with this pleasant young man for a few minutes, I can examine the ankle, make a diagnosis, and treat the problem. As I'm leaving the room, Dad asks me about his aching knee. I tell him I'm too far behind and to make an appointment.

2:45 p.m. Just like the pediatrician said, this girl sure has a bent wrist. I explain to the mother that this is not a serious fracture, but if I pull on the little girl's arm in the office, she'll scream, and it's unsafe to give a child general anesthesia in the office. Let's do it right. I'll splint the arm now so she and her mother don't have to look at it. Then at 5:00 p.m., I'll meet them at the Surgicenter to straighten the fracture under anesthesia and cast the forearm. She'll feel no pain and within an hour she can go home. Everyone will be happy. Remember, I was supposed to do a hip fracture at 5:00 p.m. at Bayview General, but we all know the hospital never runs on time.

3:05 p.m. "Hi, Mr. Crump. What can I do for you today?" I ask. He's eighty-three years young and explains that he was upstairs for his annual physical and during a routine film of his lower back, Dr. Feldman noticed that he had severe degenerative arthritis in his left hip. Dr. Feldman said it would be necessary to replace it soon and sent him down to see me. I ask him how often his hip hurts. "It doesn't. Occasionally after I've walked several miles to the store, I can feel a twinge of pain in the hip, but other than that, it's fine," he answers.

Can you believe that? Here's a guy who is sent to me because of a bad-looking hip on x-ray. It's like I tell the medical students. You don't treat x-rays, you treat people. This type of a referral embarrasses my profession. What's sad is that many of my competitors would operate on this man because it pays for their expensive houses, cars, and boats.

Wouldn't it be terrible if I put a new hip joint in this asymptomatic gentleman and postoperatively he suffers a blood clot to his lungs and dies? Why does he die? He has no pain but his x-rays look bad. This goes on in medicine all the time—unnecessary surgery, improper indications. I tell him that there is some minor arthritis in his hip and occasionally it will bother him. If it does, come in and see me and we'll try some arthritis medicine. Don't laugh at people who never go to a physician. Maybe they're not so stupid.

3:20 p.m. "Doctor, this lump on my wrist is getting bigger," Mrs. Glanville states. She has a typical volar wrist ganglion. Her family doctor told her that they hit these with a Bible in the old days, but she should see a specialist. He's right on both counts. But Bibles don't work and never did for this problem. Oh, I'm sure at times the Bible was heavy enough to bust the ganglion, but it always came back. A resident where I trained tried to stab one of these with a needle. The next thing he knew, blood was squirting up to the ceiling. He had accidentally hit the radial artery. You know, the one on your wrist where the nurse takes your pulse. Very messy.

I reassure this lady it's not cancer and if it doesn't bother her, leave it alone. If it gets too large and she wants it removed, it can be done as an outpatient procedure with a local anesthetic. She wants it removed now, so we'll arrange it and her family doctor will assist.

This is another major controversy. Should family doctors be able to assist at surgery? Do they know what they're doing? My competitors in town claim the only reason I'm as busy as I am is because I supplement local family doctors' incomes by letting them assist me at surgery. I believe the patients are always more relaxed at surgery if their family doctor is present. Many family doctors have received significant amounts of surgical training and are extremely useful assistants. They have helped me on many big cases, including hip fractures and knee and shoulder reconstructions. I know many orthopedic surgeons who are clumsier than family doctors in the operating room.

3:45 p.m. The surgery department at the hospital calls to say my hip fracture won't be going until about 7:00 p.m. But we already figured that into our plans.

4:00 p.m. This young man is alone and tells me his knees ache when he jogs in P.E. class. He states his mother wants me to check his ankles too, because last year he had one episode when they hurt. The knees look perfectly fine and the ankles are stable. The stomach is a little too big, however. But he's on a diet, only Snickers and chocolate milk for dessert. Oh, and here's the best part. He brought some x-rays for me to check. "These feet look a little smaller than yours," I joke. He explains that his mother wants me to take a look at the x-rays of his little sister's foot fracture from last year to see if I think it was treated properly by the podiatrist. I suggest he have his mother come in with him on the next visit so I can meet this inconsiderate lady.

4:10 p.m. "Excuse me, Doctor, but Dr. Split, the obstetrician down the road, is on the phone with an emergency," my secretary interrupts. You must be kidding. An obstetrician. "Hi, Buck. Listen, I have a very troublesome situation in my office that I'm uncomfortable with. I have a pregnant lady here who started her contractions this morning. I brought her into the office to see how far she was dilated and while she was climbing onto the examining table, her kneecap dislocated. She still can't straighten it and she's in my office screaming. The rest of my patients are panicking. What do I do?" he begs. I'm thinking that if she had one good contraction, the knee might unlock, but the doctor sounds desperate. "Can she get to my office so I can take a look at it?" I ask. He doesn't think he can move her, but he'll try and, if he can't, he'll call an ambulance.

4:15 p.m. I see my paraplegic patient with the broken leg. His attendant was lifting him out of bed a few weeks ago when he accidentally dropped him and his leg broke. Of course these folks have no feeling in their legs, so I have to worry about skin breakdown under their casts, in addition to fracture alignment and healing. The x-rays look fine and the skin looks good. I'm amazed how these folks can drive those battery-operated wheelchairs forwards, backwards, sideways and never touch a wall. I'm going to ask him if he's willing to give my wife some driving lessons.

4:25 p.m. "I was doing yoga today and I think I pulled a muscle in my hip," my next student-radical patient says. I can't examine people with body odor. I tell her it doesn't look too serious and she should get some physical therapy and take some medication. "I don't like to put anything foreign into my body," she says. Of course marijuana, LSD, and cocaine are natural substances with high fiber. I'm trying to figure out a way she will never return to my office. "Frequently, these muscle pulls don't respond to conservative treatment, so if it is not better in two days, come back and I'll give you a cortisone injection," I say. I was glad she had billable medical insurance because she was out the door so fast that she left only a trail of B.O. behind her.

4:37 p.m. My secretary says there is an attorney on the phone about the case that's going to trial next week and they need my testimony. I don't normally talk with attorneys on the telephone but this is a friend. "Hi, Doctor. Listen, this case involving Dr. Callroom is set for trial next week and we need you to testify on Tuesday," he says. Isn't it great that attorneys feel that they can call you, and just like that, you can drop everything? Don't they think I have any patients? "You know I can send a subpoena for you if I have to," he threatens. Attorneys with class don't do this. They know they need your help to win, so they don't antagonize you.

4:46 p.m. "Dr. Suit is on the line. He says there's a baby upstairs whose mother accidentally dropped her on the floor and the leg looks broken. Can they send her down?" my secretary asks. Great. I have ten minutes to get down to the Surgicenter to fix the child's wrist. "Tell them to hurry up," I respond.

4:47 p.m. I'd better open up some mail. That's nice. A young female patient sent a postcard from Mexico. Her knee is great and she's enjoying the sun. I would be enjoying myself, too, if I spent the week looking at the lady on the front of this postcard. I'm not complaining, though. I appreciate my many grateful patients who send cards, letters, and thank-you notes. Some bring in wine and bake me cookies.

What's this little document? Oh, come on. More nursing home visits requested by this borderline physical therapist. "Denied," I write. This patient has had enough passive range of motion to her knee. Now this looks like a request for money. The National Orthopedic Academy wants $600 this year for membership dues. For what? So the board members can fly around the country first class at my expense? But if we don't join the academy, we are looked upon as second-class orthopedists by the local medical society and hospitals.

4:54 p.m. "My goodness. What happened to you?" I say to the little baby who was dropped by her mother. The mother looks like she's in shock. Even more interesting is that the mother has a cast on her wrist. "My family doctor, who happens to be a personal friend, put a cast on my wrist for tendinitis yesterday and today, while I was picking up my baby, I dropped her on the floor," she cries. The little girl is sighing, but not in distress. Her leg looks a little rotated and shorter than the non-affected leg. This poor baby is only six months old. "Let's get a quick x-ray and see what's going on here," I reassure her. I always tell patients and their parents we will do our best to shield their private parts during an x-ray. While my technician takes the film, I hold the baby so she doesn't crawl off the table.

I'm trying to figure out why a doctor would put a cast on a wrist for tendinitis in the first place, especially when the mother is constantly picking up a newborn child and needs her hands free. You just don't treat tendinitis like this. As a matter of fact, I can't think of a tendinitis that does well in a cast. Tendinitis is from inflammation and responds to anti-inflammatory medication, physical therapy, steroid injections, and ice massage.

Well, who's the lucky guy who gets to tell Mom that her six-month-old child has a broken thigh bone? She's devastated and I'm hassled because I'm supposed to be at the Surgicenter and the nurses were nice enough to stick around until 5:00 p.m. to accommodate me. Here I sit with a situation that will take considerable explanation and TLC. But after five minutes, the mother understands that her baby will need to be in a cast from her toes to her belly button for eight weeks.

My secretary calls the Surgicenter and tells them I'm on my way. Just a little white lie. But I'll get this done quickly because my x-ray technician is such a good helper.

When I'm applying casts or suturing wounds, Sue Ellen makes small talk with my patients. I'm not good at that. She asks people, "How did you do this?" or "We haven't seen you in the office for a while, what have you been up to lately?" I just don't ask questions with the same diplomacy, even though I'm thinking the same things. Somehow my questions come out differently. Like, "How the hell did you get yourself into this mess in the first place?" or "You are such a cheapskate, how come you haven't been in to see me lately?"

We apply the hip spica cast to this poor little baby. The mother freaks out as she sees the child in this straight jacket. "How do I diaper, and what happens if the cast gets wet?" she asks. I reassure her things will be fine and we will change the cast every couple of weeks. She should call us if there are any problems. I even take a diaper and show the mother how nicely it goes around the cast. Not to worry if a little wee-wee gets on the plaster. Unfortunately, I have to explain that the two legs may never be the same length and one foot may rotate out more than the other. Of course the mother is delighted. Oh yes, Mommy's wrist. We remove the cast, I inject her tendon sheath with cortisone, and her pain is gone even before she leaves the office. She mentions that her friendship with her family doctor is over. "Good luck and don't worry," I say. And don't drop the kid.

5:15 p.m. Better get to the Surgicenter. "Thanks ladies, I'll see you tomorrow," I say, running out the door. As soon as I start the ignition, my beeper goes off. I'm put on hold by the answering service. Finally I'm told the father of the little girl I just saw with the femur fracture wants a call back, immediately. Apparently the mother went directly downstairs to a pay phone and called her husband to tell him that the little girl's leg isn't going to grow right and it will look funny. And the best news of all. He's an attorney. I'll have to call him back after surgery. I'm sure he's a very patient and understanding man.

5:27 p.m. "I know you all stayed overtime to accommodate me. I'm sorry I'm so late," I apologize. I make it up to them by fixing this fracture in ten minutes. It took longer for the anesthetic than it did for me to straighten the bone. The people here are so wonderful, kind, and good at what they do. No muss, no fuss. They get the patient in the room, do the case, and out the door.

Bayview Hospital doesn't understand this concept. Get the patient into the room, don't stop for a break. Put the patient to sleep, don't worry about the fact that, thirteen years ago, the father had prostate surgery. Fix the patient's fracture without the drill breaking, without giving me the wrong size suture, or telling me that you are out of fiberglass cast material so I'll have to use plaster today.

6:10 p.m. One of the worst things about doing surgery is you have to change clothes. Some days you practice tying your tie or buttoning your shirt three or four times. After you dress, you must dictate the operative report. "The patient was placed on the operating table in the supine position and given a general anesthetic by the anesthesia department," I state for the nine-hundredth time in my life. But, of course, this isn't always true. Sometimes we do the patient while he is standing on his head and the lady behind the salad bar in the cafeteria gives the anesthetic.

6:25 p.m. I'd better call my wife and tell her I won't be home for dinner. Remember, I have a hip to pin at the hospital. As usual, my wife understands and says if I'm hungry when I get home, she'll make me a sandwich. I thought I was supposed to get home at 6:00 p.m., have a drink, read the paper, talk to the kids at dinner about their day at school, and fix the lock on the door. So much for a normal life.

6:34 p.m. As I'm explaining to the patient's mother how I straightened the fracture, the beeper goes off. She wants to know how long the cast will be on her little girl's wrist and how I'm going to take it off. I explain to her that the cast stays on approximately four weeks and we cut it off in the office with a saw. "Although it makes a lot of noise, it won't cut her. Trust me," I say. But those are not the vibes I'm getting from her.

6:46 p.m. I'm sure surgery at the hospital beeped me so I'll just call from my car phone to see if they're ready. I'm hoping they're close to getting started. After all, it's over an hour after the time I was promised. The head nurse in surgery explains that she didn't call me, but they will be ready to go in twenty minutes. "Perfect. That's just about when I'll be there. I'm on my way," I say.

6:49 p.m. "This is Dr. Mays, did you page me?" I ask. It's the emergency room at the hospital. The doctor explains that a lady, who incidentally he has known socially in the past, tried to kill herself today by injecting paint thinner into a vein in her left elbow. "I know you're not on call tonight, Dr. Mays, but since she's a friend, I want her to have the best care available. And in my experience, you're the best," he says. That's nice. As I'm hurrying back to the hospital, I try to remember what I know about paint thinner. That's the stuff I rub on my fingers after I'm done painting. I'm really a lot smarter than people think.

6:58 p.m. "Hi, Buck, thanks for coming in," the emergency room doctor says. His friend is staring at the ceiling and crying profusely in pain. This doesn't look good at all. The elbow is very red and swollen and obviously she missed the vein and injected the paint thinner into the surrounding tissues. But she's alive. If she had injected the thinner into her vein, she would be history.

"Judy, this is not what you want to hear, I know, but we need to take you to surgery immediately and open up your elbow, so we can clean out the paint thinner before you lose your arm," I say. Already her fingers are tingling from the swelling and the pulse in her wrist is obliterated. Her doctor friend talks to her and gets the consent. Essentially he tells her she has no choice.

There isn't even a small booth to dictate a consultation note so I'll stand in the hallway with some of the intoxicated patients waiting to be seen. They hear me explain the seriousness of this injury and the terrible risks that will probably come from this paint thinner injection. "Furthermore," I dictated, "the risks of admission include death from anesthesia, postoperative infection, loss or decrease of limb function, possible need for transfusion following surgery, and the risk of AIDS." My listeners quickly began filing out the door as I finished my dictation. Was it something I said?

I remind the emergency room doctor, just in case he was too caught up in this case personally, that his patient needed a tetanus shot, antibiotics, and an IV started immediately (preferably not in the arm with the paint thinner). She also should be typed and crossed for three units of blood, stat.

7:14 p.m. Down the stairs I go to postpone the hip surgery. The operating room nurse gives me a defensive look as I walk up to the surgery desk. "Dr. Mays, you're going to be mad, but the gallbladder is going to take longer than expected and they won't be out of the room for at least another hour. They have to do a duct exploration. And what is worse, your assistant, Dr. Boat, called a few minutes ago and I told him to come right in," she says.

I ask if we could call in another team, as the paint thinner case is clearly an emergency. She says they don't have the personnel to do that. I have never heard of a major hospital with an active emergency room not having a backup emergency surgical team. I'll even bet it's against the state hospital requirements.

The elderly lady upstairs hasn't had anything to eat since six o'clock last night so I'm sure she's hungry. I hope she won't mind waiting another few hours. I'm sure her fluid requirements are so out of whack by now that it probably doesn't make any difference anyway. Not only that, hip fractures hurt like hell, which is why we fix them as soon as possible.

There's better news. The operating crew has been working six straight hours, so after the gallbladder, they need to have a forty-five-minute dinner break. But that's no problem. I'll just notify the paint thinner to stop eating its way through the patient's arm, into her neck, and to her brain.

7:25 p.m. Well, if you can't beat 'em, join 'em. I'll outsmart them and dash home for a sandwich and then come back. As I rush to the elevator to escape, a housekeeper mopping the floors asks me if I have a minute. She tells me she was in an automobile accident approximately three months ago and her neck sprain is not getting any better. Her attorney wants her to see an orthopedic specialist. Since she works in a hospital but hasn't been there long enough for medical insurance, her attorney suggested she grab a doctor in the hallway and ask him for a quick sidewalk consultation to see if she will have any long-term disability or permanent injury. That way the attorney can settle the case at a fifty-percent commission and he doesn't have to pay for records or a doctor's visit in his settlement costs. "I'm on my way out, so make an appointment in my office," I say.

7:40 p.m. As I'm speeding home, the beeper goes off. Hey, what's another call on my car telephone? Just another three or four dollars. It's surgery at the hospital saying the gallbladder case unexpectedly finished right after I left. The crew said they would forgo dinner in the interest of getting through early, so they wouldn't have to be there all night. I'm about five hundred yards from my house and I intend to go in, get a sandwich, eat it, and say hello to my kids. But is that fair to our paint thinner patient? Is that in line with the Hippocratic Oath? I grab the sandwich and head back out the door.

8:10 p.m. As I stroll into surgery, I can see Dr. Boat is angry. "Do you know I called here and they told me to come in immediately? I have been sitting here for an hour. I hate this hospital," he says. So you see, it's not only me. They treat us all the same—badly. But at least they're consistent.

I quickly explain to Dr. Boat about the emergency patient and he agrees to help me with her first. Why not? It's more money for him anyway. Two cases instead of one. The only redeemable part of the lady's plight is the fact that she has good paying insurance.

8:14 p.m. This lady is lucky. This particular anesthesiologist is terrific. He treats the patients like real people, not like objects. He talks to her and gently whispers in her ear as she drifts off to sleep. He's the best. I would let him put me to sleep.

8:25 p.m. "May I begin?" I ask. "Do what you're trained to do," the gas passer says. This case even grosses me out, and coming from a county hospital, I've seen a lot of disgusting things. The incision goes from the palm of the hand to her armpit. Cosmetically, this scar will not be attractive, but it might save her limb.

What does paint thinner do to human tissues? It looks like a combination of pus and gangrene. It's nauseating. My assistant, who's been under the weather for a few days anyway, states I might have to finish this case by myself. I clean out over fifty percent of the dead muscle tissue. We use over 10,000 cc's of solution to wash out this grunge. It's so friable that the suction tip sucks the necrotic tissue right into the hose. The skin is left wide open when we finish to allow the nasty fumes to escape. I'll bring her back to surgery in three to five days to reinspect the wound and possibly close it. The nurses all agree they're glad they didn't have dinner.

9:10 p.m. I'd better stroll into the recovery room to say hello to the lady with the broken hip and to apologize for the long delay. The beat goes on. Hospital transportation personnel were on a break, so they're just now bringing this elderly lady down, over one hour late.

My writing is so bad I had to order preprinted sheets with my standard postoperative orders. It saves time, the nurses can read it, and it decreases the chance I will be called in the middle of the night because I forgot to write for a laxative.

As I sneak into the lounge, the emergency room doctor is quizzing the rather peaked-faced Dr. Boat on the severity of the arm. I explain the thinner is mostly gone and if the tissues don't continue to decay, she may get away with a partially functioning limb. But she could require multiple surgeries and skin grafts to close the wound. I estimate at least three to four more surgeries and a very ugly scar. He thanks me very much and leaves. He looks like he cares more for the patient than he wants to tell.

9:35 p.m. Dr. Boat is sick and mad. I don't blame him. He was gracious enough to help me with the girl and now, finally, his elderly lady with the hip fracture is going to be fixed. So why is he mad? Because the hip was scheduled initially for 5:00 p.m., it's now 9:35 p.m., and we still haven't seen his patient. I don't have the guts to tell him she isn't even down in surgery yet. He tells me that the last three assists he's done have not been paid by the insurance companies. They all claim the same thing—that the procedures could have been completed by the surgeon without an assistant. I explain that even when an orthopedist helps another orthopedist, the assistant doesn't always get paid. It doesn't matter that it is safer or that the anesthesia time is cut in half because of better exposure.

9:45 p.m. Dr. Boat walks to the desk and insists on knowing where his patient is. The head nurse calls the floor and finds out that the patient has not left her room yet. "Hey," he says, "I have an idea. Let's go get the patient ourselves so we can write a nasty letter to the goddamned hospital administrator. Better yet, let's call the jerk at home and see if he would like to come in from his cozy sofa and transport the patient himself."

I can't believe it. He sounds just like me and calls the hospital operator to get the administrator on call. Then he yells at him for several minutes and then slams down the phone.

We head up to the ward to get the patient. The floor nurses object that we didn't bring a gurney from the operating room but they can see we are in no mood to negotiate. We roll this nice lady down to surgery in her hospital bed. We pass the young man from transportation coming to get our patient. He's in no hurry, carrying a can of Coke in one fist and a candy bar in the other.

9:55 p.m. As we roll the large hospital bed through the automatic doors into surgery, the supervising nurse and anesthesiologist look up in amazement. "What happened to transportation?" the anesthesiologist asks. You're looking at it, sports fans.

10:10 p.m. "Dr. Mays, can you tell me what suture you would like to use? Your preference cards are lost," the scrub technician says. I've only been operating here for five years, but it is probably too much to ask that the nurses know my suture preference. Besides, tonight we have nurses brought in from the registry. That means they don't know a thing about this hospital or me, and, in this case, very little about orthopedic surgery. I become concerned. The patient is in the room, but where is the x-ray technician? In all the excitement, our supervisor forgot to call x-ray. I've already fetched the patient so I may as well go tell the technician we need the image intensifier machine now. This isn't in my job description.

10:16 p.m. It sure smells good in x-ray. They're all sitting around eating pizza and I'm hungry. Jokingly, they offer me a piece if I don't need their help tonight. They already saw that I had a hip fracture to do. The guy who normally helps us do these fractures is here, but he gets off at 10:30 p.m., so we'll have to take a new lady. She says she has done only a few hip fractures but claims she knows the equipment well. I explain that the patient's x-rays from yesterday aren't in surgery. They promise they'll find them and send them down. I grab a piece of pizza and run.

In the surgery lounge, Dr. Boat is yelling at the administrator who, unbelievably, came in from home. "How would you like to spend the whole damn day in your office, then sit around here all night waiting for a case to start because you cheapskates won't pay for a second surgical team? We had to go upstairs to get our patient because your great transportation workers were unavailable to do their jobs," Dr. Boat rages.

Hospital administrators can usually talk their way out of anything and they have excuses for everything. He explains a second surgical team is not cost-effective because there is too much overtime involved and forty percent of the time the team isn't needed. Furthermore, the transportation people are part of the union, so they must have a stipulated number of breaks or else the hospital is subject to fines. I suggest we put the administrator on the fracture table, point the cost-effective x-ray beam at his microscopic nuts, and radiate the bimbo with 5,000 rads, so he can glow in the dark at tomorrow morning's administrative staff meeting!

10:45 p.m. The anesthesiologist puts a spinal needle into our patient's back and numbs her fractured hip. It takes only a minute because he's slick. He told the lady before he stuck the needle in her back that she would feel a little mosquito bite. With some anesthesiologists, it feels like a shark bite.

She's all set and ready to go. The x-ray technician positions her machine. As she prepares to take an initial film, I remind her that everyone needs a lead apron on before she shoots a picture. After thirteen exposures we have the x-ray tube finally positioned right.

I'm reviewing the surgical equipment with the scrub nurse. She admits she hasn't done a hip fracture for three years because she does urology at the hospital where she usually works. That reminds me to urinate before this case starts.

11:05 p.m. As the nurses begin washing the hip, I go tell Dr. Boat we're ready to go. He's still "chewing" on the administrator. I love it. I always thought that if we could fire the top ten administrators at the hospital, it would run more efficiently, the doctors would be happier, and they'd have enough money for a second surgical team at night.

11:10 p.m. We finally begin. This case, which was put on early this morning for a 5:00 p.m. start, is finally beginning at 11:10 p.m. I make the incision. Minor bleeding is controlled. Retractors are placed in the wound and we position a guide pin into the hip. The hole is drilled, the screw is placed up the neck, and the plate is secured to the pin and bone. Final films show good position of the screw and plate. The hip looks great. I'm sick of hearing that orthopedists are glorified carpenters.

Isn't it incredible? We waited over six hours to do this case and it took us eighteen minutes, skin-to-skin, to perform the surgery. The patient lies around in pain the entire day without food. The doctors are exhausted, the nurses are hungry, and the system stinks.

11:30 p.m. As I enter the surgeons' dressing room, I see a note on the door with my name on it. The nurses on the ward are concerned about the amount of drainage coming through the dressing of our last patient and they would like me to stop by and check it before I leave the hospital. With a little luck, she will be asleep and I won't have to hear about the suicide attempt.

No such luck. She is awake and looks depressed. I tell her not to worry about the prognosis tonight, but to get some rest and we'll talk in the morning, when we are both fresh. But wait, good news! She has feeling in all of her fingers. Miraculously, she is moving them all.

11:42 p.m. I'd better quickly stop by my office to get the charts and x-rays for tomorrow's five surgeries. One rewarding thing about going home at this time is that there is no traffic. But my wife and kids are asleep and that is not rewarding. My eight-year-old daughter left me a note: "Daddy, we miss you. Don't work so hard."

12:05 a.m. Finally, I climb into bed after eating an apple and looking at the sports page. It's hard to sleep with all of these problems on my mind, but I'm so tired I drift off.

12:57 a.m. The phone rings. It's the answering service to tell me that the nurse taking care of the paint thinner patient wants to talk to me. "Dr. Mays, I'm sorry to bother you, but I got to work late and I didn't get a chance to hear the nurses' report. It seems that this lady is having a lot of drainage," she says. I'm so mad I want to scream. I take a deep breath, count to ten, and then I scream. "I was just up there a few minutes ago and saw the dressing and it looked fine. If you'd get to work on time to hear the report, you wouldn't have to bother me!"

That's one interesting thing about the night shift. They have to be up anyway, so if there is any question at all, call the doctor. By all means, don't attempt to use your head.

1:25 a.m. I'm still awake, wondering when the phone is going to ring next. Even more stimulating is the thought that I may get to do the same routine again today. Remember, I have to fix the spaghetti lady's hip. She's on at 5:00 p.m. Does this sound like a broken record?

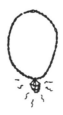

26. The Ultimate Diamond

As MY practice began to flourish, I was making an enormous amount of money but enjoying life less. But hard work meant big bucks. That was important to me. I was frequently at the office, in the emergency room, or in the operating room until midnight. I enjoyed being busy and popular in the medical community, to a fault. Even when it was Dr. Laddie's weekend to cover the practice, I took my own calls and wore the beeper the entire time.

I was only free from these chains when I went out of town. I felt no one could do it better than I, so I made myself available around the clock. Mr. Orthopedics.

This was further compounded by my associate, who hated to take calls and responded accordingly. He answered his beeper if and when he felt like it. Sometimes this was within an hour or two and sometimes not at all. This, of course, made patients very unhappy, especially if a patient's injury involved a great deal of pain and swelling.

In one case, a boat trailer ran over a patient's foot while I was in Florida with the football team. Dr. Laddie had decided to enter a golf tournament and cover calls from the course. He responded about four hours later because he didn't believe that he should be disturbed during the competition. He simply turned off his beeper. The patient waited an hour and then went to the emergency room because her foot was swollen and bleeding. I could not dictate how Dr. Laddie treated his own patients, but I would not allow him to treat mine in this fashion.

It was the Monday following this episode that Dr. Laddie and I first exchanged harsh words. It was prompted by the verbal lashing the patient's mother had given me upon my return. She said, "Get yourself another associate or we'll get ourselves another orthopedic surgeon." She was right.

It was a shame. Dr. Laddie was addicted to golf like an alcoholic was addicted to liquor. He had to have it at any cost. He couldn't live without it. Golf made him act unprofessionally and irrationally. Worse than that, it had cost him his profession, his livelihood, his reputation. His ability to earn a living was destroyed and he didn't realize it. The words of the local pediatrician on my first day in Bayview kept ringing in my ears: "If you're going to succeed in this town, you'll need to find a different associate, one that's available when we need him."

Dr. Laddie played golf at least three times a week. He often played when he said he wouldn't. How did I know this? I lived a few blocks from his country club and drove by several of the holes each day. On Saturday or Sunday mornings when he was supposed to be covering the practice, I would spot him on the second tee or the sixth fairway. I wasn't spying. I was just on my way to make rounds at the hospital because I knew he wouldn't. I had an associate in name only.

I have to admit, though, as the years went by, I often thought about Dr. Laddie's philosophy. He claimed that physicians made themselves too available to the public, that most of the calls at night and on the weekend could wait. He frequently laughed at a doctor's need to wear a beeper every second of every day to be totally available. Patients could call any time of the day or night for any reason.

More often than not, he was right. Probably eight out of the ten calls I received on weekends or at night could have waited. Like the patient who ran out of medicine on Saturday and was too dumb to figure out on Friday that this would happen. Or the mother who called on Sunday to say that her son had hurt his knee last Wednesday, but it had continued to swell over the past three days so she thought she should call.

I finally figured out a way to reduce the number of these calls. I had my secretaries give out an information sheet to all my patients when they came to the office. They read it while they waited to see me. It told them about me, my training and my background. It also explained office policies such as requiring payment at the time of service and filling prescriptions only during office hours. The information sheet further explained that I was happy to receive calls for acute injuries after hours but the exchange was instructed not to call me for anything other than emergencies after hours or on the weekend. This worked well and I received fewer unnecessary calls. My mood improved dramatically; if only I had thought of this sooner.

If I were going to work hard, I wanted to get something in return. My father always told me, "It's the smart man who works for his money and then lets his money work for him." There were fortunes in medicine to be discovered and I stumbled onto one thanks to my bad temper, Dr. Quackmont, and Mark Chump.

I was seeing a local judge for an acute back strain that he had suffered while lifting the convertible top onto his Mercedes. He could hardly walk. I examined him and it seemed like a severe muscular strain. I wrote him a prescription for muscle relaxants and suggested he see a physical therapist for deep heat and massage. As I filled out a referral form for All Sport Physical Therapy, he inquired, "Is there a place I can go after hours or on the weekends, since I'm on the bench all day?" I told him I would make inquires and get back to him. I pondered his question and thought about All Sport. I sent all my patients there because Dr. Quackmont was the medical director and I felt an obligation to him for helping me get started in Bayview. Remember, he promised to get me privileges at the university. One hand washes the other.

I had my secretary call All Sport to see if the judge could be seen evenings or on the weekend. She was told there were no evening hours and the receptionist laughed when asked about weekends. That amazed me since most of my patients worked during normal business hours, and it was difficult get away to go to physical therapy.

I called Mark Chump, the head physical therapist. He responded, "We have always felt that if a patient needed therapy badly enough, he could take time off from work." Now I was getting angry.

I called Dr. Quackmont. He was very supportive of my idea, but added that Mr. Chump made policy concerning therapy and hours. Even though he was the medical director he said he couldn't intervene. I was appalled. I sent them fifteen to twenty cases a week. You would think that if I wanted personal limousine service to and from my office they would oblige. I guess not.

I continued to see the rest of my patients while formulating a plan that would turn out to set a precedent in the medical community. As I was driving home that night, it suddenly came to me. Why was I sending all of my patients out the door when I could establish my own physical therapy facility?

The ultimate plan was forming. I would open a physical therapy center in my office that would function when I was out of the office. I would see patients during normal business hours and my physical therapy unit would be open nights and on the weekends. All I needed was a therapist and some equipment. I became more excited when I realized this would help cut my overhead expenses by at least thirty percent.

My last hurdle was to discuss this with Dr. Laddie. He was very sensitive about the office because he had the lease and paid for all of the improvements himself. In addition, I had become much busier than he in a very short time and I was clearly using more of the space. It was hard to predict what he would say. On the one hand, if it cut both of our overhead expenses, he would rejoice. But if therapy patients were in the office when he wanted the space, he would probably object. I had the answer. I'd offer Dr. Laddie a piece of the action.

The next day I presented my offer. He had no objection to the idea as long as the therapy hours didn't interfere with his practice. He questioned how professional the office would look with a large knee rehabilitation machine in the exam room and a whirlpool in the cast room, but he said he was willing to give it a try.

Here was the amazing thing. He thought there were already too many therapy facilities in town, and he seriously doubted that another one would be successful. He wasn't interested in a partnership. I couldn't believe it. We could refer five to ten patients a day, just between the two of us. How could it not turn a profit? So be it. I'd reap the benefits alone.

I placed an advertisement in the newspaper for a therapist and ordered all the standard therapy equipment, including weights, hot packs, ultrasound, whirlpool, and a knee machine. I became more and more excited. I took out a fictitious name permit and the Bayview Orthopedic and Sports Therapy Center was quickly becoming a reality.

I received a call from Mark Chump, who had seen my ad for a therapist in the local paper. I'd never known him to be so polite. "Dr. Mays, sorry to bother you at your office. I was hoping we could work out something to your satisfaction in order to better accommodate your patients. Do you have any time to get together and chat for a few minutes?" he inquired.

I asked him if he had decided to stay open at night or on the weekends. He replied that he had consulted with the other therapists and they all decided that was not the direction they wanted to take at this time. I told him these next few weeks would be very hectic for me and I would get back to him. I meant I would send him an invitation to the opening.

I found that hiring a therapist was more of an obstacle than I had anticipated. It was well known in medical circles that the National Association of Physical Therapists looked down on therapists working in therapy centers owned by physicians. They felt physicians were padding their own pocketbooks at the expense of physical therapists, who were finding it tougher to succeed in private practice.

But I couldn't believe that all therapists felt the same, especially if they needed a job. This was a unique opportunity for someone to work in a private setting with their weekdays free. I felt sure that someone out there wanted to work closely with an orthopedist to learn the business.

I was right. I found a therapist, Cookie, within three days. She had previously practiced in a hospital and wanted a smaller setting with a greater variety of patients. She was aware of the dictum by the physical therapy association, but it didn't concern her. I told her if I ever referred a patient to her inappropriately, to please let me know.

We agreed on salary, made a few equipment modifications, and shook hands. We would open in two weeks and decided at first she would see only my patients. If it worked out, we would have a big open house and announce our unique operation to the entire community.

This was clearly looking as though it could be a great achievement. I had a sign made for the door, and printed special physical therapy prescription pads on bright yellow paper. My secretary agreed to do the billing for a minimal increase in salary. She began calling insurance companies for therapy contracts. We encountered little resistance and almost everyone commented, "What a great idea."

The day came. We opened on a Monday night at 5:00. I had already made several referrals during that day, so we were off and running. Cookie took extra time with the first patients so we could assure success. My secretary and I waited with anticipation.

By the end of the evening, we had seen seven patients. After they were gone, we cracked open a bottle of champagne. Cookie was excited about the patients and felt all of the referrals were appropriate. My secretary said the insurance billing procedures were easy and we billed $1,250 for the first night. I began to realize the potential of this business on my way home and nearly ran off the road.

Over the next several months, I felt like a mastermind. The therapy schedule was full and appointments were getting hard to come by. I frequently had to go into the emergency room at night and I would stop by my therapy unit to chat with some of the patients. They thought it was great that they could go to physical therapy and see their doctor too. "Hey Doc, look at how well this knee is moving. I think I'll be ready to ski next week," one said. "Oh, Dr. Mays, I'm so glad you're here, because I'd like to get a refill on my medicine." This was better than a phone call.

Occasionally, there were small problems. Sometimes Dr. Laddie would come in after hours. Instead of his peaceful office, he would find pure pandemonium. There would be three people in the waiting room, two in the exam rooms, and one lying on the x-ray table icing his knee. Cookie would have her nightly snack of soda water and fruit scattered all over the famed couch in our private consultation room. This annoyed Dr. Laddie.

The most difficult thing for him was realizing that he had made a major mistake. The therapy was busy and successful, and it was happening right in front of his eyes. Every day. He complained how dirty the rugs were because there was so much traffic in the office. I did one better and replaced the carpets. The therapy business could afford it.

Our charges were impressive and our overhead was minimal. It wouldn't be long until our collections would be substantial. After our first quarter, I was in disbelief. No wonder the National Physical Therapy Association was on the warpath. These damn therapy units generated a lot of income. This little idea of mine was putting so much money on the books, I could hardly believe my eyes. Even after paying the therapist a generous salary and contributing a large chunk to office overhead, there was $75,000 left over. I paid off all of the equipment and bought a new computer to handle the extra workload.

I had found a pot of gold by accident, by doing the right thing for my patients. And even better, word was spreading around town that I had a therapy service with evening and weekend appointments available. Cookie was acquiring a great reputation for her low back massages.

We had an open house catered with all the trimmings. I invited every potential referrer in town. When it became so busy that people were waiting two to three weeks for an appointment, we hired an aide to help Cookie, expanded the weekend hours, and added two afternoons a week when Dr. Laddie and I were off. The Bayview Orthopedic and Sports Therapy Center began to make a fortune. I started to feel like I had robbed a bank.

Six months after we began, I received word that All Sport was out of business and that Mark Chump had moved out of town. That was another thing my dad told me, "What goes around, comes around." And it did. I fantasized that I would open up more therapy clinics and hire Mark as an aide. But I really shouldn't be bitter toward him. If it weren't for him, I wouldn't own Bayview Orthopedic and Sports Therapy Center.

Things continued to fall into place. During the final year that the Intruders were in business, I convinced Dr. Laddie that our satellite office in Casa was inadequate because we had no x-ray machine and the owner of the building would not allow one. In the back of my mind, I was saying to myself that this office was too small for a physical therapy clinic.

We decided to look for space in the nearby town of El Rancho. We found a beautiful new building that was centrally located. I designed the new interior space, complete with x-ray equipment and a physical therapy center. The Bayview unit had plenty of money to finance the entire operation.

At the end of the football season, as many had predicted, the league "went belly up" and the Intruders folded. They were broke and let everyone go. But wait a minute. What about my contract?

I went to the general manager with a plan. I told him that I had $8,000 remaining on my contract but because the Intruders were out of money, I would accept all of the equipment in the training room as payment in full. I explained I was trying to set up a new physical therapy practice in El Rancho and this would help me get started. He thought a minute and came to the same conclusion I had. The equipment in the training room was worth a lot more than $8,000.

But he reasoned that I had done a good job for the team and a lot of personal favors for his very sick parents when they came to visit from New Jersey. He also knew he would have to go to considerable trouble selling the equipment anyway. He agreed to let me have the goods. I thanked him profusely and arranged for a friend with a large truck to meet me in an hour, before the general manager changed his mind. We loaded the tables, ice machines, and rehabilitation equipment into the truck and drove straight to a storage outlet to store it for two months while the new clinic was being built.

The horror stories I had heard about construction companies were awful. The Clapp Company, building my space in El Rancho, was no different. Politics reared its ugly head as I was told I had to use this company by the people renting me the space. The company was owned by the chairman of the board of trustees at Bayview, Mr. Clapp, and the hospital had an interest in this building. But why should I be worried about Mr. Clapp's capabilities? The hospital had only fired two presidents in four years and was $10 million in debt. The morale of the physicians at Bayview was at an all-time low. Other than that, he ran a great ship.

Three months after the promised date, the space was finally finished and it looked pretty good. Now all we needed was the furniture and we'd be in good shape.

I remember calling the decorator about ten days before we were scheduled to open, wondering if the furniture would arrive on time. She had already forgotten about my order and had moved on to her next job. But she agreed to check it out and call back. She learned that the examining tables and waiting room furniture were coming from Massachusetts on a truck that had left three days ago. The only problem was that they hadn't heard from the driver in three days and the police had found the truck abandoned near Chicago. The good news was that the furniture was still on the truck.

While we waited for the furniture, I was contacted by one of the radiologists at Bayview General, Dr. Lanzoni, whose group had long wanted to establish a presence in El Rancho and wondered if I had any extra space they could lease. He was favorably impressed with my building and the reputation I had established as a businessman.

I said I was going to have my own x-ray facility, but he assured me that his group was interested in attracting the larger studies from local doctors like barium enemas, scans, etc. He assured me they had a deal for me that would be beneficial to all.

He met me at the El Rancho office the next day and we looked over the space. He commented on several occasions what a great job I had done designing the space and how it was perfect for a small radiology operation. With a few minor changes in electrical needs and floor plans, they were ready to sign on the dotted line. I must admit I was very proud of the entire space, most of which I had designed myself with the help of an architect. Even without the furniture, it looked impressive. The space was flexible enough to accommodate almost any type of practitioner that wanted to lease some part-time space and help defer costs. Dr. Lanzoni assured me he was the group's spokesman and that everyone was enthusiastic. We agreed on rent and improvements and shook hands. We had a deal. Over the next ten days, the contractors made the improvements. All our furniture arrived and the place looked spectacular. We were ready for business.

Or at least I thought so. Two days before opening, I received a call from Dr. Dung, the chief radiologist at Bayview. He asked if he could run over to my office and have a quick word with me. When he arrived, I noticed he seemed uncharacteristically shy. He softly said that all the radiologists had met this morning and everyone was shocked at the commitment that Dr. Lanzoni had made to me. He continued that things were moving faster than they had expected and that the group did, in fact, have an interest in coming to El Rancho. But the timing wasn't right and he wondered if there was any possible way they could get out of the deal.

I asked Dr. Dung if he had any idea how much I had spent upgrading the space to their specifications and the number of people I had turned away who were interested in the space. He apologized again and said that we all had to continue to work together in the community and they certainly didn't want me as their enemy. They were willing to compensate me for my trouble. Now they were beginning to talk my language.

I leaned back in my chair and shook my head. I told him if I didn't have $25,000 in twenty-four hours, I would file a lawsuit against his group for breach of contract. He thought this figure was too high but promised to present it to his group. I reminded him that Dr. Lanzoni had repeatedly told members of the medical staff that they were opening an office in El Rancho and I was sure there would be no shortage of doctors around who would testify to that fact.

Later that day, Dr. Volve, another radiologist in the group and a neighbor of mine, called and asked if he could stop by my house on the way home. I told him not to come by unless he had the check for me in the full amount.

As I expected, he showed up at 8:00 p.m. sharp. He asked if we could chat alone for a few minutes. "Frankly," he said, "the group thinks Dr. Lanzoni went far beyond the power we had given him and for that we are all very sorry. We all believe you are the major force in orthopedics in Bayview and we sincerely hope to establish your trust again. We need to go forth and we don't want you as our enemy. We want to be able to feel free to contact you in the future if we have another business proposition. The group feels $25,000 is excessive but we are willing to pay that to call a truce and put this behind us." He handed me the check, smiled, and left. I had won that battle, but little did they know that was merely round one in this title fight.

For several days I was angry, but the reality of the situation took precedence. I had just made $25,000 very easily. Because of them, I had upgraded my x-ray machine considerably. Even better, I found two more tenants within a week. We would all share the rent and expenses, and it turned out that this operation would cost much less than my space in Bayview. And it was twice as nice. It was designed by me, for me.

There were other slippery doctors who wanted to sublet my space. A group of family doctors in my building in Bayview approached me about renting space. Their spokesman, Dr. Alta, was a grey-bearded punk who walked around the corridors of the hospital with his head held high like a peacock. He was active in political circles but had a small patient following, so he had to work part-time in hospital administration to make ends meet. He asked how much the monthly rent would be in El Rancho.

I was suspicious of him from the get go because he never sent me any patients. I told him $500 a month and $5,000 for leasehold improvements. He had already seen the office and was very impressed. He agreed the price was reasonable but said his group was currently cash poor because they had just taken in a new associate. I asked how much he could afford. He said "$200 a month and no leasehold improvements." He tried one final ploy, "We see a great deal of orthopedics in our practice and we could send you patients in place of the rent."

I was born at night but not last night. I knew his group was friendly with Dr. Small, so I told Dr. Alta his offer was out of the question. "What guarantee do I have of your support in the future?" I asked. He said he would give me his word. The word of a friend of Dr. Small made me want to gag. I told him to keep his referrals and off he went. Neither he nor anyone in his group has sent me a case since. That was the amount he had sent me before this conversation.

The bottom line was that the office in El Rancho opened on schedule and it was an instant hit. Word spread quickly that we had a gorgeous office in a prime location with plenty of parking. We were busy in a hurry and the physical therapy took off as it had in the main office, with several other doctors in the area sending patients.

What a refreshing change from practicing in Bayview, where many patients wore sandals, had poor medical insurance and poor hygiene. People in El Rancho dressed well, paid cash or had good insurance, and bathed regularly.

Dr. Laddie just sat back in awe as I continued to expand my empire. He made comments to me time and again that he might be ready to invest in the physical therapy business now. But he was too late. It bothered him tremendously that the ten patients a week he sent to my therapy units were adding to my pocketbook. I assured him that these patients were helping to defer our overhead expenses. But he knew the truth. I was just getting richer.

The physical therapy businesses were completely legitimate. All the patients needed therapy and our therapist was of the highest quality. The patients were happy and Cookie was happy. And I was ecstatic. She kept saying how she had never seen such a variety of orthopedic problems. She treated people with tennis elbow, low back pain, shoulder bursitis, neck sprains, and hip tendinitis. She loved them and everyone seemed to get better.

You can imagine all the stories floating around Bayview about me now. The entrepreneur of medicine strikes again. Many doctors began saying that I was more worried about my pocketbook than my patients. Dr. Small called me "the Donald Trump of medicine."

Soon I noticed that internists were joint-venturing and opening up laboratories together. And, the best compliment of all, Dr. Small's group opened their own physical therapy center. The same guy who had called me "the Donald Trump of medicine." I told him one morning before a hospital orthopedic meeting that I was disappointed it had taken him so long to follow suit. I always tried to establish rapport with my competition.

I branched into consultation when an urgent care doctor from a nearby town came to see my new clinic. He asked me to design and joint-venture a physical therapy center for him. I was concerned because our personalities were very different. Also, many practitioners in his area thought he was running a makeshift operation and providing minimal care to patients. Four doctors had left him within one year.

I offered to design the office and oversee the therapy operation for an initial fee of $5,000 and then a percentage. He agreed to this quickly after he reviewed the revenue reports from my two facilities. I designed the office and the entire production was ready in six months. We both did well.

Then I met a truly terrific physician, Dr. Gold. He had referred a patient to me with a knee problem which ultimately required surgery. Dr. Gold assisted me with the operation. While we were sitting in the surgeons' lounge waiting to start, he began quizzing me about my therapy businesses. I could see he was favorably impressed. He complained, "I wish family doctors could participate in ventures like that. You surgeons make all the money while we just scrape by, even though we send you our cases." He began to chuckle and said, "Why don't you open another therapy clinic in Bayview and let all the family docs invest? Then you'll be the busiest orthopedist in the West." Why the hell didn't I think of that?

We were called to surgery and continued the discussion as we scrubbed our hands. But I already had decided in the last thirty seconds that this idea would become a reality. I damn near cut myself twice during the surgery, anticipating my next move with Dr. Gold. The plan started taking shape as I closed the skin.

The therapy operation in my Bayview office was getting too busy and we were ready for expansion. Dr. Laddie was getting angrier about this money machine right under his nose. I decided to close the therapy unit in my office, move it a few blocks away into a brand-new medical building, and joint-venture with several referring doctors in the community. I envisioned a few of Dr. Small's most loyal referrers jumping ship.

I announced my intentions to several physicians and we held our first meeting. Over thirty people attended. I was careful about what I handed out on paper as I knew somewhere in the room was a spy for Dr. Small and his partners. I decided to meet with all prospective investors individually. I made Dr. Gold a general partner and my liaison to the local primary care doctors. We had them eating out of our hands. They couldn't wait to sign up. I began designing my fourth clinic, meeting daily with the architect and the builder because I wanted this to be my best effort yet. It was on the main thorough-fare through Bayview and local doctors would pass by every day.

We had several meetings with our limited partners and this time Dr. Laddie climbed aboard. Several goals were set by the partnership and Dr. Gold and I let it be known that no one would be "carried" by the rest of the investors. We wrote into the contract that if a doc's referrals were significantly below the average, the general partners had the right to buy out his interest. We knew that legally this was shaky but we didn't want anyone receiving equal dividends and con-tributing nothing to the business. We opened and within days were the talk of the town. Dr. Small was seeing red by this time and told a mutual friend that "someone has to stop Dr. Mays, he's a maniac." I was just getting started.

Dr. Gold and I examined the books after three months of opera-tion. We were seeing an enormous amount of patients, but our collec-tions were not that good. A local physical therapist contacted me and said how impressed he was with our therapy setup. He wanted to know if I was interested in selling and mentioned that he had his own billing computer software. His accounts receivable were impressive. I told him selling the business was the farthest thing from my mind.

But then an idea struck me. What were the major hassles in my therapy practices? Finding employees, billing, collecting, and man-aging were the biggies. So I asked him if he would be interested in a fifty-fifty arrangement. He seemed puzzled. I went on to explain that we had the one thing he needed, patients. I proposed he manage the operation, hire and fire the therapists, bill and collect the money, and our group would continue to own the business and pay the rent. At the end of the month, we would split the money collected fifty-fifty. He said it sounded good but he'd have to run some numbers off and get back to me.

The next day he called and approved the deal. His charges for services were thirty percent higher than ours but after checking them out, we found they were within reason. His collections were also far better than ours. He knew the right codes and responses to billing questions from insurance companies, and our receivables improved considerably. Another whim of mine was paying off.

Unfortunately, a few of our partners were not sending the patients they had promised. Some hadn't sent one in three months. So Dr. Gold and I did the unthinkable. We kicked three of them out. We showed them the figures of everyone else and obviously they were not supporting the business. We bought them out at fair market value. Dr. Gold and I were criticized by these three for several months, but business is business. I felt bad about leaving them out in the cold, so I referred them to Dr. Small as another possible joint venture specialist.

Dr. Small was known as a great judge of character anyway. He took another questionable resident into his orthopedic practice. Dr. Baldi was interested in bone tumors. He was very outspoken and never achieved much of a reputation as a surgeon. When he came to town, he immediately announced that he was the most brilliant and educated orthopedist in the area. He went straight to the surgery department at Bayview and talked the operating room supervisors into buying totally unnecessary equipment to "update" our antique collection. He convinced the hospital administration that without these new toys, they were liable. He insisted on using ultraviolet light during total joint replacements, even though there had never been an article in the literature that proved its effectiveness. The nurses were afraid to go in these rooms for fear of being burned, and the anesthesiologists had to draw straws to see which one got to wear the space suit for a day.

He was an obnoxious little brat and his wife divorced him soon after his arrival in Bayview. So Dr. Baldi started romancing every nurse in the hospital. He finally settled on a physical therapist, Mildred, and began learning the tricks of the trade from his mentor, Dr. Small. Mildred was not appreciated at Bayview General Physical Therapy, so while I wasn't watching, she was sent by Dr. Baldi to apply for a job at our therapy unit. You guessed it. She was to spy on the operation so they could learn how I made so much money. But I caught her and got my people to fire her. This was apparently no problem as her attendance record was horrible.

There were things that were as predictable as the sun rising in the morning. A few months before his orthopedic board exams, Dr. Baldi asked my opinion about preboard study courses. I told him I hadn't attended any. But I began thinking about the Boards and how humble you must be to pass. Any examiner who senses cockiness or conceit will fail you on the spot. Dr. Baldi didn't disappoint me. The hotshot failed the Boards. Bad public relations for the practice. Both he and Dr. Small disappeared for several weeks following this defeat. I just sent my sympathy card to their office.

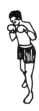

27. Put Up Your Dukes

IT WAS only a matter of time until Dr. Small and I came to a show-down. As he had pointed out the day I arrived, there was room for only one orthopedic group in Bayview—his group.

From the outset of my appearance, Dr. Quackmont promised to help me obtain privileges at the university student health center, where he was the senior athletic physician. He told me he would keep hounding Dr. Small, his good friend of twenty-five years, until I was offered a position. But things took a peculiar turn as the months rolled on.

One day at the country club, I ran into Dr. Quackmont. This was now two years after he had assured me of the position. I took this opportunity to once again ask him, "Any idea what's happening to my application for a spot at the student health center?" He looked around to make sure no one was listening and then asked me to sit down. Noticing his peaked face, I asked if anything was wrong. He responded, "I feel responsible because I persuaded you to come to this community and I promised to help you obtain privileges at the university. I've discussed the situation with Dr. Small again and I was outraged at his response. Because I feel obligated to you, I'm going to tell you exactly what he said, but if you ever tell anyone I told you, I'm going to flatly deny it." I agreed and asked him what Dr. Small had said. He continued to look down, embarrassed to look me in the eye. "Dr. Small said that he would never take a Jew into the orthopedic department at the university as long as he was chief." Then he stared at me, obviously sharing in my discomfort.

I told Dr. Quackmont that I was shocked but I had heard remarks before in the community about Dr. Small's anti-Semitic behavior. I regained my composure and asked him what he would do if he were in my shoes. He said he didn't know what to say. He tried to convince me that I had done very well on my own and that I didn't need the university position to succeed. I sensed there was something else he wanted to say, but he got up and headed into the locker room, barely saying good-bye. He looked ashamed.

A few months later I discovered the remaining pieces of the puzzle. As I was dictating charts in my office, Dr. Laddie came into the room and remarked, "Did you hear the news about your good buddy, Dr. Quackmont?" He smiled and continued, "Dr. Quackmont is financially strapped and can't pay for his big new house up in the hills overlooking Bayview, so he's taken a position as a sports medicine consultant in Dr. Small's office." How could this be? Dr. Quackmont, my father-in-law's close friend at the country club and my co-sponsor into the club. I had been so naive. Sure, it all made sense to me now. Dr. Quackmont merely encouraged me to come to Bayview because he was my father-in-law's friend. He never had the slightest intention of helping me get into the university. I had referred at least fifteen patients a week to Dr. Quackmont's All Sport Clinic so the place would survive and he could keep his meaningless job. I received virtually no referrals from him. I should have realized then, but I had trusted this dishonest son of a bitch.

All along, I had been a good boy. I hadn't made any waves. I only begged once a year for an explanation about my university privileges. But once a year, he could dodge a bullet and lie. He and Dr. Small had conspired all along to keep me out of the student health service. Why? Because I was too good. I would take over most of the orthopedic surgery at the university when the students found out there was a better alternative to Dr. Small and his flunkies.

Things backfired on the enemy when I opened my own physical therapy unit and All Sport went out of business. Dr. Quackmont was fired from his position and didn't have a job. How would he pay for his fancy new house and his country club dues? Along came Dr. Small, who hired him on one condition. Dr. Small didn't want to hear anything more about me getting privileges at the university. Lay it to rest. Dr. Small was the boss now.

These two were capable of even more dishonesty and fraud. You might ask how a family doctor, like Dr. Quackmont, could work in an orthopedic office. He wasn't an orthopedic surgeon. But why not? Dr. Quackmont advertised as an orthopedic surgeon in the yellow pages even though he had not had one day of formal training in orthopedic surgery. It sounded fraudulent to me.

Enough was enough. The picture was crystal clear to me. Since I had arrived in town, two other orthopedists had joined Dr. Small's group and both of them were granted immediate privileges at the university. The orthopedic department there was a closed shop. It was a public institution for which I paid taxes and I wanted in, now. I called Dr. Small and very politely asked him if he would meet with me for a few minutes so I could get his advice on a matter. I knew this would work because he was the great godfather figure and he loved people asking him for advice.

We met in the doctors' lunchroom at 5:30 p.m. the next day, and I shook his hand and thanked him for coming. He sat in a chair against the wall, ready for the firing squad. "Well, how can I help you?" he asked. "Dr. Small," I apologized, "I've had a problem for the past few years and I haven't known where to go with it so I figured I would go straight to the 'horse's mouth'" (even though I meant ass). "You see, Dr. Small, I was brought to this town by your friend, Dr. Quackmont, because of my keen interest in sports medicine, and he had assured me I would be able to work with the athletes at the university. He told me, being your close friend and all, he would talk with you and I would be allowed on the orthopedic staff. As you may recall, I mentioned my interest to you when I first came to Bayview." I could see he was starting to get very nervous and his face became colorless. "In any event," I said, "you have chosen to admit two more orthopedists to the staff at the university, who just happen to be in your private practice, without even considering my interest. So, you see, Dr. Small, I called you here tonight to say that you have exactly forty-eight hours to give me privileges at the student health service or I will file a lawsuit against you and the university."

I actually jumped as Dr. Small leaped from the table. He pounded his fist on the table and was enraged. "Let me tell you something, Dr. Mays," he yelled, "I'm an institution in Bayview and have been for over thirty years. No one can sue me. If you think our relationship has been casual up until now, you haven't seen anything yet." He stormed out of the room and slammed the door. He hasn't spoken a word to me since. As promised, I filed the lawsuit forty-eight hours later.

Word of the lawsuit spread one hundred miles wide, and faster than a doctor-nurse affair. The reaction was initially mixed. Many of the old-timers in town who were friends of Dr. Small were outraged that a doctor would sue another doctor. Other physicians around the community applauded my courage and said they, too, had tried getting privileges at the university but the "good buddy" system had prevailed. It was obvious that I had started a civil war in Bayview. Depositions began and records were subpoenaed.

The situation became even nastier. Dr. Small and his posse sat at their Monday morning meeting plotting ways to get rid of me. They decided to start by having Dr. Stalin bring up charges against me at the hospital quality assurance committee. He looked for the slightest mistake on any of my charts to make me look bad. An elevated temperature in a postoperative patient. Normal for other doctors but a complication for Dr. Mays. He found a hip fracture patient who had required a blood transfusion, even though virtually all hip fractures need blood. But the consent for transfusion was lost (in Dr. Stalin's pocket). He was slick. He waited until Dr. Laddie, who was on the committee and my only defense, was admitted to the hospital for more treatment. Several members of the committee told me it was obvious that Dr. Stalin had a personal vendetta against me and not to worry. He could only convince them to write me a nasty latter. Nice try, though.

Next Dr. Small's group arranged to have another of their new associates, Dr. Baldi, sit on the surgical review committee for the Hopeless Health Plan in an attempt to deny my requests for surgery. That way, I wouldn't be quite so busy. But it turned out that he was having too many personal problems and he missed so many committee meetings that all of my requests were granted. I just kept operating. I know Dr. Small wondered what had gone wrong with his latest ambush when Dr. Baldi showed up at the Surgicenter with only one case scheduled and I had six. Embarrassing. Back to the drawing board.

I was on call one evening when I was summoned to the emergency room to see an elderly lady with a fractured hip. She mentioned that she had had previous knee surgery by a Dr. Small. I suggested he be called to care for her but the patient pleaded with me. She said that Dr. Small was insensitive and too old to operate. And she couldn't stand the other partners in his group who had made rounds on her the last time. So I agreed to fix the hip. Dr. Small, as was his custom, went to the orthopedic ward each morning and spied on the new patient charts so he could keep close tabs on who was busy. He noticed the name of "his" patient and became incensed that I had operated on her. He cornered me while I was making rounds and jabbed his finger in my chest. He said, "What the hell do you think you're doing operating on one of my patients? This will come up before the surgery committee." I explained what the lady had said, but he only grew more outraged. He told me I did it just to spite him and he was sick and tired of my interference in his life. Little did he know this was just batting practice. The game was yet to begin.

During these stressful times, Dr. Small experienced chest pain on several occasions and had to be admitted to the hospital for tests and placed on heart medications. But I don't hit people when they're down. I wanted to help so he would be healthy for the upcoming trial. So I called the cardiac intensive care unit and left instructions for the nurses to call me for Dr. Small's bowel-care orders.

28. Is the Grass Always Greener?

MOST doctors base their hospital practices primarily in one location. This means we admit most of our patients to one hospital and do the majority of our surgery there too. In the case of Bayview General, most of us sit around complaining about everything from the wards to the operating rooms.

The wards are understaffed, with many nurses who speak poor English and are slow to respond to patient needs. The operating rooms are so disorganized that patients have to wait six to eight weeks to have an elective case done. The turnover time in the rooms between cases is so bad that we frequently have time to wander over to our offices and see several patients before the crew has cleaned the room for the next case. At times I dreamed about working at another hospital. Bayview General is a pit.

One day, one of my patients had a special kind of medical insurance that required me to operate at another hospital ten miles away. I already had privileges there, but seldom used their facilities. I scheduled this knee case and, when the day came, I dashed over about a half hour early.

I had no idea where to park, let alone where the operating room was located. I had heard that the hospital was like a maze. Also, I wanted to make sure that the nurses knew what sort of equipment I would need so I wouldn't be waiting for my tools during surgery. A surgeon should always do this but seldom does.

I didn't want to be late to my first case at a new hospital. That would leave the staff with a bad impression. Doctors always think they have a built-in excuse to be late, wherever and whenever they want. We can learn to be on time just like normal folks.

I rolled into the operating room about twenty minutes early and introduced myself to the lady at the front desk. As I was inquiring where I could change into my scrubbies, there was some confusion in the hallway. Moments later a large woman approached me and introduced herself. "Hi, Dr. Mays," she said, "I'm Mrs. Hite, the head nurse. I'm sorry to tell you this on your first visit but your case is going to be delayed. The gynecologist in the room you will be using inadvertently penetrated the bowel during some minor female surgery and we had to call in a general surgeon to help out."

She directed me to the men's changing area. As I strolled down the hallway, I wondered if this was just bad timing or if every hospital was the same. Damn! I changed my clothes and headed for the coffee room to have a doughnut. As I picked up the sports page, an elderly gentleman approached. "Hi, I'm Dr. Nitol. I'm an anesthesiologist here. I don't believe I've met you before. I'm sorry you picked such a bad day to come here. We don't normally make this kind of a first impression on a new doctor. I heard Dr. James was revived right away and I'll bet they'll be out of there in a few minutes." "Who's Dr. James?" I questioned. "Oh, didn't you hear?" he said. "Dr. James is the gynecologist who was doing an oophorectomy (ovary removal) on a lady in your room and he punctured the bowel, so Dr. Ileus, a general surgeon, came to fix it. When Dr. Ileus arrived in the room, Dr. James fainted cold on the floor. We had to revive him while Dr. Ileus closed the lady's wound."

I giggled and thought this had to be a joke. As Dr. Nitol and I exchanged the usual pleasantries of where we each worked and lived, there was a knock on the door. Mrs. Hite entered and said she had good news. Since my room was going to take a long time to clean because of all the instruments that were required on this rather unusual case, she was going to move me to operating room three across the hallway. Another orthopedist was just closing a tiny finger wound. I should be able to start in fifteen minutes. I thanked her profusely and assured her I was enjoying my conversation with Dr. Nitol.

She thanked me for my patience and said she wished all doctors were as patient as me. Another nurse came in to tell her to get to room three immediately. Did she say room three? That's the room I'm supposed to be using. I went out to see what was happening. "What the hell's happening in room three?" I asked one of the nurses.

They were just taking a man off the operating room table after a finger operation and as they were moving him onto the recovery room gurney, they accidentally dislocated his shoulder. They had to reanesthetize him to relocate his shoulder. "But I think they have it back in the socket now," she smiled.

I never thought in my wildest dreams I would ever wish I were back at Bayview General, but it crossed my mind. I shook my head as I went back for my fourth cup of coffee. In the doctors' lounge I met Dr. Ileus, who began telling of his woes in the punctured bowel case. As Dr. Nitol and I listened intently, we heard an announcement over the intercom paging any anesthesiologist stat to the recovery room. Dr. Nitol leaped out of his chair and Dr. Ileus followed close behind, wondering if it were his patient. I followed thinking that this was fast approaching a legitimate episode of MASH.

Everyone was huddled around the patient who had a bandage on his finger. The recovery room nurse told me that this patient just had a respiratory arrest. "They had to intubate him but he seems to be waking up now," she muttered.

Mrs. Hite was coming toward me. "Well, Dr. Mays, believe it or not, we're almost ready to go with your knee." I thanked her and went back to the coffee room. And guess what? Within ten minutes she entered the now crowded doctors' lounge to tell me my patient was in the room, on the table, and ready to go. Granted, it was one hour and ten minutes later, but I had to admit it was pretty damn exciting around here.

I entered room three and greeted my patient. I also introduced myself to the surgical scrub technician, the circulating nurse, and finally to the anesthesiologist. He was getting his gas machine organized so he didn't have too much time to chat with me. Ten minutes later, the patient was asleep and I was told to go scrub my hands while they prepped the patient's knee. After washing my hands, I entered the room, gowned and gloved, checked the instruments, and draped the patient's knee in the usual sterile fashion. After all the arthroscopy tools were hooked up and ready to go, I glanced at the head of the table and asked the anesthesiologist if I could begin.

As I did, I could hardly believe my eyes. The anesthesiologist nodded yes to me as he held a mask over the patient's mouth with his left hand and another mask over his own face with his right hand. I looked on in complete disbelief as the scrub tech asked me if I was okay. I turned to her and asked, "What's the deal with the double-fisted gas passer at the head of the table?"

She whispered that this particular anesthesiologist was allergic to the anesthetic gases given to the patient, so he had to oxygenate himself as well as the patient during the case. I took a few moments to gain my composure. Was this really happening? Amazingly, I finished this fairly easy, straightforward case in twenty minutes. Both my patient and the anesthesiologist woke up.

My patient got to the recovery room with all of his limbs intact. As I wrote the postoperative orders, I promised myself I would take back everything I had ever said about Bayview General.

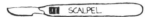

29. The Surgicenter

EVERYTHING about the Surgicenter was right. It was located on a busy street with easy access to the rapid transit system. The architecture was modern and the interior was comfortable and classy. Patients had the feeling that they were not in a hospital. They were not surrounded with sick terminal patients but rather with healthy, active citizens just there for a quick, in and out, safe procedure.

The staff was polite and efficient. The rooms where the patients waited with their families before surgery were quiet and well furnished. Once the patients awakened after surgery, they were taken to a discharge lounge to be with their families. Here they could chat or rest quietly until alert enough to leave.

The Surgicenter was not well received by all the physicians in the community. The old timers, like Dr. Small, were opposed to any kind of change. They didn't want a facility that would compete with Bayview General, the hospital where many had practiced for thirty years. It didn't matter that the facility was nicer and better equipped for outpatient surgical services. No change was good change.

But the docs in the area who were busy and needed to keep a more rigid schedule were impressed. We knew if we had surgery scheduled at 7:30 a.m. at the Surgicenter, we would cut at 7:30 a.m. At Bayview General, a 7:30 a.m. time meant we might start at 8:15 a.m. if all went well. Since time was money this just wouldn't do.

At first the Surgicenter was not busy, because it took time for people to get their secretaries used to scheduling cases away from the hospital. Once they did, they were "hooked." It was easier and the staff scheduling the cases was far more polite than at the hospital. If a requested time was not available, the Surgicenter would find a way to accommodate you.

The medical director, Dr. Snootful, was a gem. He was older but wiser. As an anesthesiologist he was the best. Surgeons knew that with Dr. Snootful at the head of the operating table the patient was safe. He made the cases go quickly, one after the other. Once his patient was awake and comfortable in the recovery room, he headed for the pre-op room to get the next patient ready for surgery. Seemed simple.

This was a concept the anesthesiologists at Bayview General could not grasp. Once they finished a case, it was off to the coffee room for a doughnut or down the street to the BMW dealership to take their cars for repair. To hell with the next patient or the entire schedule for that matter.

The Surgicenter was heaven for the surgeon. It was one of the few places where I was honored to be on the board because I cared about the place. I loved working there and my patients loved being operated on there. But once again I found myself a fish out of water on the political scene.

My first encounter with the board took place when an ownership share in the Surgicenter unexpectedly became available with the death of a local doctor. Dr. Snootful strongly suggested we sell it to an ENT surgeon, Dr. Tripter, who had promised he would use the Surgicenter exclusively if sold the share. The rest of the board nodded their approval. "Bullshit," I said. "There are many members of the community who have been coming to this place for months and they want the share too. Let's sell it to someone who has been supportive." The prevailing feeling on the board was that although I had a good point, the surgeons already using the place were going to continue doing so and this share was a way to entice new blood.

I conveyed to the board the many discussions I had had with members of the community concerning Dr. Tripter. Several sources had stated that he was all talk and very few people took him at his word. But the board thought I was sulking and ignored me. They approved the sale of the share to Dr. Tripter.

At the board meeting three months later, I asked the administrator how many cases Dr. Tripter had done since purchasing the share. He wasn't sure, so I asked the chairman to excuse us so we could look it up on the computer. The final score in a three-month period: one case.

I politely told the board that they had reneged on their fiduciary responsibility. I never let them forget that. In a way it served a purpose. Over the next three years, when I felt strongly about issues, I simply reminded them of the Dr. Tripter caper and collected on my debt.

One nurse, Morski, was a big favorite of mine. She worked as a circulating nurse in the operating rooms. Previously she had been the supervisor at the county hospital and had a wealth of experience. She came to the Surgicenter to semi-retire, giving her more time on the golf course and on the ski slopes. When the head of surgical services left the Surgicenter and Morski was asked to take over, she refused. We were desperate.

The Surgicenter was starting to get busy and this vacancy was potentially a major setback. The last thing the board needed was a long search process for a new supervisor. So I took Morski and her husband out for a nice Japanese dinner and begged her, as a favor to me, to take the position for one year. She reluctantly agreed and assured me this would cost me, big time.

The staff was ecstatic over her change of heart and Dr. Snootful agreed there was no stopping the Surgicenter now. Morski collected on her promise within a few weeks. She said she needed someone on the patient care committee. And I was her man.

After several meetings in which we reviewed postoperative complications and patient satisfaction responses, there appeared to be only one major problem. Many of the patients had complained that they were being discharged too early, before they were ready to leave the premises. They had been forced out because it was getting late in the day.

After the fourth complaint I suggested we call the patients to see if they remembered a face or a name because I was highly suspicious of one of the recovery room nurses. Brenda was noted to be very abrupt and rude. Some of the nurses who knew I was on the board had taken me aside and told me of the problem. We guessed right. It had been Brenda all along. I suggested to the administrator that she be fired because she did not exemplify the professional spirit of the Surgicenter. He agreed.

The next day Dr. Snootful pulled me aside and said he would consider it a very personal favor if I would back off on my criticism of

Brenda. He didn't go into detail, but he reassured me that Brenda knew she had a problem and she had agreed to counseling. He promised to oversee her progress and I noticed tears in his eyes. I felt bad and wondered about their relationship. Since I really liked and admired Dr. Snootful, this didn't seem to be too much to ask. I agreed.

Brenda was better for a while but then started to lose her temper repeatedly. I heard of these episodes but never saw them firsthand. Morski said she was still uncomfortable around her. Then one day as I was operating on a knee, Brenda entered the room to tell me I had forgotten to write out a prescription for pain pills. I told her I would do it as soon as I finished this case. She commented, "My God, the great Dr. Mays made a mistake."

All the eyes in the operating room stared at each other. My assistant and two nurses commented that someone had to do something about this witch. After the case I stormed into the administrator's office and said if she was not fired by the end of the day, I would cancel all future surgery at the Surgicenter. She was gone by noon.

The last black mark against the Surgicenter was the most upsetting to me. It concerned Dr. Misled. Initially Dr. Snootful had been able to handle most of the anesthetic chores because business was slow for a few weeks. As the schedule became busier, he was in need of another anesthesiologist.

I told him about a lady, Dr. Misled, who was outstanding with patients, pleasant to the surgeons, and liked to work quickly, which would fit right into the philosophy of the Surgicenter. He interviewed her and said she would do fine. However, he seemed troubled that she was a woman and made no formal long-term commitment to her.

Things went smoothly for several months, but Dr. Misled would frequently show up and sit around the entire day and do only one case. Dr. Snootful stole most of the cases instead of spreading the wealth. But Dr. Misled was a good sport and waited patiently.

As we got busier, Dr. Snootful said it would be difficult to take any vacation with just two anesthesiologists on staff. He asked Dr. Misled if she had any friends who might want some part-time work. She talked to a male colleague, Dr. Nic, who started spending a few days a week at the Surgicenter to get acquainted. This worked well for several months and Dr. Snootful took some time off. Drs. Nic and Misled were getting more cases.

One night at home I got a call from Dr. Misled which shocked me. She said Dr. Snootful had offered Dr. Nic a full-time job and never mentioned it to her. She confronted him and he said he had had no idea she was interested in a full-time position and never thought to ask. He insinuated that because she was a woman, she didn't need full-time work.

I was irate. I had helped Dr. Snootful once, but this was war. He wouldn't get away with this. And I felt guilty. I had brought Dr. Misled to the Surgicenter, where she had sat and cooled her heels for months just so the place wouldn't lose any cases.

I confronted Dr. Snootful the next day in person, as I wanted to look straight into his eyeballs. He rationalized his move by saying he thought we would lose Dr. Nic to another hospital if he didn't hire him full-time. Secondly, Dr. Snootful said he had questions as to the competence of Dr. Misled as an anesthesiologist. But why hadn't we heard of his concerns before? Why did he allow her to practice there for months if he questioned her capabilities? I was livid. I began phoning other surgeons who used the Surgicenter and they were all appalled at the news. Dr. Snootful spent the next few weeks "dodging bullets." No one was satisfied with his explanations.

A weekend board retreat took place a few weeks after this insult. I insisted this topic be discussed. To my surprise everyone on the board criticized Dr. Snootful for his handling of Dr. Misled. He reacted by standing up and yelling at me with a clenched fist. He finally sat down when he realized the entire board was furious. He had embarrassed himself beyond belief and hadn't recovered by the next day, missing that day's meetings. Upon our return to Bayview he avoided me. Dr. Nic did all my cases, which hurt Dr. Snootful financially, as I was the busiest surgeon there. Since then, our relationship has been casual, at best. Dr. Misled took a job elsewhere.

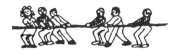

30. Medical Insurance

WE HAVE all heard that you get what you pay for. Well, this applies to medical insurance too. Today you have several choices of health insurance programs. Of course you can choose to have no insurance, which makes more sense than meets the eye, except if you have a catastrophic medical problem.

There are large health maintenance organizations (HMOs) with which we are all too familiar. Patients in great numbers belong to these because they are the cheapest health insurance plans and are often paid for by employers. Again, if you are healthy, these HMOs are adequate.

The drawbacks, however, are numerous. Typically when phoning the HMO you get a recording: "The orthopedic clinic is closed today. If you have an emergency or a problem that needs attention immediately, go to the emergency room."

So you go to the emergency room, where there are usually thirty people waiting. If you want to wait, it is usually three to four hours to see the doctor. That's assuming the doctor doesn't want x-rays or laboratory studies. If he does, give it another two hours. This is because when you get to the laboratory or x-ray areas, there are usually another twenty people waiting.

You must remember, too, that when you are seen it will be only by an emergency room physician who is not a specialist in any area of medicine. He will probably give you temporary relief until you can get an appointment in the appropriate specialty clinic over the next several days. If your problem is severe, then the on-call specialist can be reached, but usually not for an hour or two.

Of course if you decide that the scene in the emergency room is too dreadful, you can go home in pain and call the clinic in the morning. This is fun, too. Routinely you get another recording, and then finally an advice nurse. She may tell you your injury is nothing to worry about, which will give you great confidence, I'm sure.

If you're lucky, she will fit you into the clinic schedule that day. Likely it will not be with the doctor you request. You see, there is always one doctor in each department who is required to have a few openings in his schedule so that acute callers may be seen. This is required by law. Occasionally, if you know the system, or have brought bagels to the doctor or his nurse in the past, or your husband coached the doctor's son or daughter in Little League, you can get in to see your favorite physician. But you have to know the special telephone number or private line of this person, who gives it out only to special customers.

Private insurance is the most expensive, but it is the best. You can choose your own doctor, who is always on call, twenty-four hours a day, to see you. You can normally see a pediatrician, a family doctor, an internist, or an orthopedist within an hour, at any time. They also know you better.

If you were referred by a primary care physician, the specialist will respond quickly. That is good business and the way of private practice. The specialist wants the business and is complimented, in most cases, that another doctor thinks enough of him to refer the case. Any private doctor will most often meet you at his office or in the emergency room.

In addition, I tell my patients, if you hurt yourself on the weekend or at night, call me. I can save you time, money, frustration, and incompetence. I'm not saying that all emergency room doctors are incompetent. Actually most are very good. But they don't know as much about orthopedics as I do, so why not go to a specialist?

Emergency rooms have gotten away from their original intent. Patients should go there only with life-threatening situations. But thousands of people are using emergency rooms as outpatient clinics. Then they are angry when the appropriate treatment is not administered. A patient stubs his toe and is wondering if it's broken. Another's back has been hurting for several weeks and it is not improving, so he thinks he should come in. What is an emergency room doctor going to do in these situations? Temporize, and suggest the patient see a specialist in the morning. This is not necessary, because private insurances will cover legitimate specialist visits.

Medicare is for older patients. It is important to take care of our elderly. Medicare doesn't pay the doctor very well, but most of us realize we are going to be old one of these days, so we treat the elderly the way we would want to be treated.

The controversy surrounds whether the doctor will accept assignment. This means the doctor can take what Medicare pays and be happy, or turn around and bill these patients for the remainder of their balances. This issue has brought out some of the real intelligent business minds in physicians as well as some of the more compassionate ones.

My associate, for instance, states, "I'm not going to let anyone tell me how much I can charge or be paid, young patients or old." In principle, he may be right. But practically speaking, he doesn't understand. First of all, many of these people don't have any money, so you can send them bills every month until you're blue in the face. You can call them on the phone or even turn them over to collection agencies and they still don't have any money.

If they have any money, we all know that the doctor is the last one to get it. "Doctors make too much money," my elderly neighbor says. She further adds, "Doctors are too rich and they don't need the money." If a patient decides to pay you, it is frequently one to five dollars a month until the balance is paid off. By this time, the doctor is normally eligible for Medicare himself. Many doctors don't consider how many hours their secretaries spend trying to collect these often small accounts. I would rather my girls spend their time scheduling new patients with private insurance or satisfying the ones I have. Collecting on delinquent accounts is difficult enough without trying to collect from the elderly.

Medi-Cal, the insurance for the indigent, is terrible for the doctor, but great for the patient because it's free. Many doctors, especially the good ones, don't take Medi-Cal. If a referring doctor asks me to see a Medi-Cal patient, I do it. I don't mind doing my part for these people, but I can't allow my practice to have an excess of these non-paying customers. Medi-Cal pays practically nothing to the doctor and is a bother to process, creating endless amounts of paperwork. I pay dearly for cast materials and x-ray film, but Medi-Cal does not give adequate compensation for them. The patients are incredibly unreliable and, more often than not, are late for their appointments or don't show up. Finally, they can be noncompliant. They lose their prescriptions so don't take the medicine you have prescribed to help them.

There is also the Happy Health Plan. This insurance plan allows you to choose your own physician. Of course they aren't honest enough in their ads to tell you that the physician has to be chosen out of their provider book. They don't tell you that the physician had to pay a large sum of money just to have his name printed in the Happy Health Plan Directory.

The Happy Health Plan tells their customers that their plan is the greatest. They say that patients don't have to fill out any papers or pay doctors any money. For only a few bucks you can get your prescriptions filled. What they don't tell you is that they contract with only a few pharmacies in each city, so you might have to travel several miles to get drugs.

Now how about the quality of care? If the Happy Health Plan starts running low on cash, what is the best way to control the problem? It's obvious — to them. Find the procedure that is costing the most money and don't allow that procedure to be done without going through a special committee. Ignore whether or not the procedure is indicated, or if it is in the best interest of the patient. This way the Happy Health Plan can control spending and filter a few cases through once a month and the other patients can wait.

One of these unfortunate patients was a young man who owned a construction company and did a lot of lifting and climbing on ladders. As I examined him, he complained that his knee would frequently give out and lock on him. One time he felt he was about to fall off a ladder when his knee buckled on him. He had all the typical findings of a torn cartilage in his knee, so I requested permission from the Happy Health Plan to do the surgery. I tried to obtain authorization. Because of the anticipated delay, my office scheduled the surgery for three weeks down the road. My patient was not thrilled. We also ordered a special magnetic resonance study on the knee to help convince the Happy Health Plan that he needed surgery. The price of this test, for a diagnosis I already knew, was $800.

It was on this occasion that I was first informed that all patients needing arthroscopy of the knee would have to have their cases reviewed by a special committee to see if the procedure was indicated. When my secretary told me of this, I called Dr. Rolly, the medical director, and asked, "I wonder if I could find out exactly who is on this committee deciding if I may do arthroscopy on my patient." The response would soon be heard throughout the medical community. I was told the committee was made up of three doctors: two family doctors and a chest surgeon.

So, let's review this in our minds before we hit the ceiling. Two family doctors and a chest surgeon were sitting in judgment of an orthopedic surgery procedure with which none of them had had any experience. I asked Dr. Rolly why I was not on a committee to decide whether a heart surgeon could do a coronary artery bypass surgery? Or why was I not sitting in judgment of the general surgeon who wanted to take out a gallbladder? Why was I not called when the diabetic specialist wanted to give one of his patients a shot of insulin? I hung up on the bastard.

It was obvious what was going on. The Happy Health Plan was running out of money, so the review committee delayed these cases hoping that the patient would either get better or go somewhere else. One week passed and I didn't hear from the authorization people, so my secretaries called the Happy Health Plan. They assured us that they knew of our request and would let us know shortly. Three weeks later, the day before the surgery was scheduled, we had still not heard. Did this omnipotent committee not have time to review the case? My patient's knee continued to give out and lock on him and probably some irreversible arthritis had occurred already.

I got on the phone to call Dr. Rolly, but he was in another meeting. I asked to speak with his administrative assistant and was told that she was out for the rest of the afternoon. So I informed the administrative secretary of the dilemma and I said if I didn't hear from them by the end of the afternoon, I would assume it was all right to go ahead with the procedure. She agreed and promised to get back to me by 5:00 p.m.. This was around 2:00 in the afternoon. Of course we didn't hear a thing the rest of the day.

The following day, I explained to the medical director at the Surgicenter about the authorization problem and that we had not officially heard from anyone giving us permission to proceed. We both agreed that it was in the best interest of the patient to operate and we assumed that the authorization would be forthcoming. The surgery was performed and took all of fifteen minutes to find a large tear in the patient's cartilage which was removed easily. The patient left the Surgicenter without crutches two hours after the anesthetic wore off.

A week later I received a letter from Dr. Rolly reprimanding me for performing an unauthorized procedure and advising me that another committee would be formed to determine if my membership in the Happy Health Plan should be terminated. I explained all this to the patient and he was incensed. The referring doctor wanted me to take legal action. All I wanted was to make the patient better.

Your choice is very clear with medical insurance. If you like the luxury of private insurance, you will have to pay more, but you will get better service. Health maintenance organizations (HMOs) are usually inexpensive and are paid for by employers, but they are incredibly insensitive and unresponsive to the patient's needs, especially in an emergency. Expect to talk to a lot of answering machines and to see several different doctors for the same problem. Prepaid health plans allow some flexibility in choosing a physician but are very politically administered. Should you consider having no insurance at all? It makes more sense than meets the eye, especially for young people. The question you must ask yourself is, "How lucky do I feel?"

31. Reimbursement for Services

WHEN I went to the supermarket this week, I got some milk, soft drinks, potatoes, bread, and a few other items. The bill came to $27.42. I paid in cash, although the lady in front of me wrote a check. In other words, money talks and bullshit walks.

In the medical business, only about one-third of your patients, if you are lucky, have private insurance. For the majority of patients, their insurance companies must be billed. You are not allowed to collect any money up front, even if the patient wants to pay, and that's damn unusual.

All doctors' offices are different when it comes to private insurance. Some offices bill the patient's insurance company and then the patient is billed for the remainder not covered. In this case, the doctor gets the privilege of acting as a bank, except we can't be open from 10:00 a.m. to 4:00 p.m., Monday through Friday. We can't even have the stuffy lady behind the counter scold you for not filling out the deposit slips right. But we can lend you the money for your office visit until your insurance company decides to pay, which is frequently six to eight months after they receive the bill.

Other doctors' offices, if the insurance is appropriate, make the patient pay up front at the time of the visit, and if the patient wants to get the money back, he can fill out the insurance forms and send them in to his insurance company. If they are not filled out correctly, which is the case ninety percent of the time, the patient can go look in the mirror for someone to blame. The doctor is essentially saying, I want my money now and if you want yours, fill out the stupid insurance forms. They are only two pages long.

Another way, which we use, is a compromise. If possible, we charge the patient up front but we bill his insurance company for him. This pacifies the patient because even though he has to put up the money initially, we can fill out the forms more proficiently than he.

Occasionally, even when you know what you are doing, the forms come back. Sometimes the insurance companies send forms back just to prolong payment. That way they can keep the cash longer to invest. In this scenario, the doctor's office computer-bills the insurance companies repeatedly.

When an insurance company gets your bill, they first look to make sure that the person is a member in good standing. Frequently a member is denied through computer error or misspelling of a name or numerous other ploys which allow them not to pay. For those members in good standing, the benefits of the patient are checked. Are the services that the physician performed covered under this plan? Was the visit necessary? You may be asking yourself, do the people asking these questions have any training to make these decisions? In our experience, usually no.

Okay. The insurance carrier decides that the patient is a legitimate member and is fully covered. Now, it says on the bill that he was seen in the emergency room at ten o'clock on Saturday night for a fractured forearm. The emergency room doctor looked at the patient's arm, ordered an x-ray, saw that the fracture on x-ray was bad, and called the orthopedic specialist. The insurance company classifies it as emergency treatment and pays. What do they pay? The emergency room doctor bills for a consultation in the amount of $75 and is paid $45. The radiology department sends a bill for $50 and receives $27.50. Also, the Ace bandage and splint are billed at $40 and $16 is reimbursed. Remember the supermarket? This isn't fair.

The insurance companies got together and decided they would deduct a certain percentage from the charges to make ends meet. The doctor does have an option. If he doesn't like it, he can shove it!

But let's not let this interfere with patient care. The bill so far is $165 and the insurance company pays $88.05. But wait a minute. What has been accomplished? The patient is still in pain with a fractured arm, and has not seen a specialist yet.

The patient and his parents are in the cast room. They appear quite angry because they have been there for three hours. I explain how sorry I am but I was just called about ten minutes ago. I set the fracture quickly and rush him over to x-ray to make sure the bones are lined up. They are, and off they go, very appreciative that something finally happened.

I saw the patient, anesthetized the fracture area with some local injecting medicine, reduced the fracture, casted the forearm, and got an x-ray. This took twenty minutes. My secretary bills $100 for an emergency room consultation and $350 for the anesthesia and reduction. The insurance company pays $62 for consultation and $175 for the anesthesia and reduction. X-ray bills for a postreduction film and gets paid the same as before. The emergency room bills $60 for the cast material and gets paid $20.

The radiologist comes in the next morning at 9:30 a.m. and reads the films. "There is a fracture of the distal forearm which is angulated at about thirty degrees. A postreduction film in the cast shows adequate alignment of the fracture fragments." He bills the insurance company $50 and gets paid $37.50.

If you paid careful attention, the radiologist got paid the highest percentage and contributed absolutely nothing to the care. The patient had been seen, treated, and released without the help, advice, or expertise of the radiologist.

This is reimbursement. The average time it takes to collect on these bills is between three and six months. Many of our accounts are over a year old with no activity. The whole damn thing is depressing.

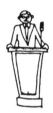

32. Medical Education

PHYSICIANS, more than any other group of professionals, are not only expected to keep up on their specialties, but are monitored by federal and state agencies. Most professionals just read a journal or attend a yearly conference and that's that. But not so in medicine.

There are several ways you can get your medical education credits. You can read medical journals. Most of the articles have absolutely no relevance to the everyday practice of medicine, but that doesn't make any difference. Just read and get your credits, so you can say you've learned something.

Another way to prove your knowledge is to teach. You can be a professor at the university and get credit for instructional hours. Personally, I have always enjoyed exchanging knowledge with students and residents because I think it is a unique learning experience for both parties. I always learn from the residents because they can quote all of the latest articles in the literature. My experience is something about which they cannot read.

The problems that arise, however, are many. In order to teach, you usually have to go to the university or to a special hospital. As you might imagine, this is very inconvenient and almost impossible to do regularly if you have a busy practice. Emergencies take precedence and office hours frequently get extended. The only way around this is to simply block out an entire morning or afternoon of your weekly schedule. The way I get around this inconvenience is to tell the university that I'm happy to teach, but that the students or residents must come to me.

Another problem with teaching is that the full-time professors at the university are very protective of their students and residents. They must be considered the primary teachers at all times. If the students or residents begin to like the private practicing physicians, we usually receive a polite letter stating, "We very much appreciated your participation last semester, but due to scheduling conflicts, we will not need your services next year."

The full-time staff hear that I am a sensation with the arthroscope and normally do six cases in a morning when it takes the same amount of time for the faculty to do two cases. The bottom line is that residents who train solely with the medical school faculty will be technically far inferior to residents who have spent time with private practicing orthopedists. In fact, the best orthopedic programs are those that are supervised by orthopedists who are part-time university employees and part-time private practitioners.

And what about the students? Things have really changed since my days in medical school. I made rounds at the hospital a few months ago with a group of third-year students on their surgery rotation in orthopedics. Seven students showed up. Four on time, two within a half hour, and one over an hour late. There were many excuses, like having to run back to an apartment for orthopedic textbooks, and having to change a cast on a patient in the clinic. There were three girls and four boys. Three of the boys were in golf shirts with no ties or white coats. All three girls wore pants and only one wore a white coat. They had been on orthopedics for about two weeks. It was really depressing. They had been taught no principles.

The final straw occurred around 5:00 p.m., when one of the girls asked me how much longer I thought we would be. She said she had to catch a ride home with a friend who always got off her pediatric rotation at 5:00 sharp. One of the guys added that the reason he wanted an orthopedic rotation was that he had heard he would never have to stay later than 5:00. "Hey, folks, I'm here for you, so you let me know when you're bored and I'll get out of your hair," I responded.

Let's call a spade a spade. The students in medical school today work less than I did. With the amount of facts you need to learn in a four-year period, they simply can't pick up all the information needed to practice good medicine. The students are not any smarter than we were and they don't read any faster than we did. The future is looking bleak, but with all the other problems, like decreasing incomes, increasing politics, and federal and state intervention, it's a mess anyway.

So if you don't like to read much and teaching is not your bag, what's left? Well, you can always go to a seminar. This is an area in which I have a great deal of expertise. As most of the public is aware, doctors frequently head off to medical seminars held in beautiful places. It has always been questionable whether the doctors even showed up for the course or merely signed in and left.

My first exposure to medical seminars was when I was a resident. Because of my sports elective and involvement with a professional football team, I was asked to speak at a new course. It was being held at Bent Tree Lake, given by our own university and chaired by Dr. Spud. He told me that I was the first resident to ever give a lecture. I was happy I attended because it taught me right away, from square one, how not to run a course.

Because Dr. Spud was a full-time faculty member and had to run the program through the school of medicine, there was a limit to what he could be paid. So rather than have the university make a lot of money off his course, he decided to ask every one of his friends to give a lecture. It was politically expedient. All of his friends would owe him a favor.

Why should the university make money off Dr. Spud? They already paid him far less as a professor than he could have made doing the same surgeries in private practice.

The following year I was asked by Mrs. Rody, who worked in the university's medical education department, if I was interested in chairing a course on sports medicine. Quite an honor for a resident to be asked to chair his own course, I thought. We discussed the program and basically they wanted my name on the brochure with my professional football affiliation in big bold letters. They said I would have to choose my faculty from the university and I could select very few outside speakers. I told them no deal. I had experienced the canned talks of university professors and they weren't the least bit stimulating. If I were to be the chairman, it would be set up the way I wanted with my topics and my faculty. We ended up compromising and I asked two people from the orthopedic department at the university. Besides, I still had to graduate and I might need a job one of these days.

Next we sat down to do the budget. Because of protocol in the university system, I couldn't be paid any more than Dr. Spud. But I insisted on the same honorarium and, much to my amazement, she agreed. Since it was the first year and a relatively new subject matter, we decided to budget for fifty participants and hold the course close to home.

The last major task was to design an attractive brochure that would catch the eye of prospective participants, and I accomplished this on my own. I depended on the department of medical education to mail the brochure to the appropriate people.

Ninety-eight participants signed up and the course was a great success. For the most part, the lecturers were very good and the evaluations at the end of the seminar were terrific. We had minor mistakes, like not enough food during the breaks. One of the presenters read his notes and was boring. But overall the program was a success.

Mrs. Rody had a postcourse lunch and said, "I think we made more money on your course than on any other university-sponsored course this year. But that's not for publication or we'd have several hundred jealous faculty members on our hands." I thought about it and she was right. The tuition for the course was $300 and we had attracted forty-eight more participants than budgeted. That was almost $15,000 and they only gave me $500 plus expenses for masterminding this operation.

The next year I was chief resident. When they approached me about doing the course again, I insisted they restructure my salary. They paid me as both a faculty member and as an organizer. Basically, they doubled my salary and expenses. We held it at Bent Tree Lake and I kept most of the same faculty. We budgeted the course for 100 participants and 144 signed up.

I recognized that this could be a very profitable business. Our first year wasn't just luck. If you put together a good solid course with good faculty and held it in a nice place, it meant success. I was determined before I left the university to learn as much as I could about mailing lists and accreditation. I figured I could run these courses yearly, on my own.

I was not really interested in doing this just for the money. Rather, I had put together a product that was well liked and well attended and it seemed foolish to stop at this point. I had the formula for a successful and meaningful experience for practitioners wanting to learn about sports medicine. I knew I could make enough money to break even, and I would get a nice vacation out of it too. There was plenty of time for play and relaxation because we had only four hours a day of didactic material. We usually lectured in the mornings from 8:00 a.m. to noon and then took the rest of the day off.

I took a giant gamble the third year. I decided to hold the course in Hawaii. Everyone involved with medical education programs discouraged me from doing so. Yes, it was a great place, but it was expensive to fly the faculty there, and it would be difficult to make money. Of course it was much more expensive for participants to get there, especially if they wanted to bring their families. There was a big chance that fewer people would sign up. But I had never gone along with the status quo. I invited fewer faculty to cut down on overhead and lowered the tuition.

I put up $15,000 out of my own pocket to design and print the brochure, buy the mailing lists, and pay for postage. I was getting nervous. The brochure had been out six weeks and I had gotten only three positive responses. Where did I go wrong? Was all the negative feedback I had received earlier correct? Registrations started to slowly accumulate. I ended up with 175 sign-ups. After all course expenses, which included several faculty dinners and a mai tai reception, I netted $5,000. I put the money in a money market account in the course's name and set my sights on next year. Back to Hawaii.

I knew I had conducted the most financially successful sports medicine seminar in the country. From the detailed evaluations I collected at the end of the course, we did a good job of teaching, too. I was absolutely amazed to see that most people actually came to all of the lectures. I insisted the hotel give me some perks if I was bringing over a hundred people to their property. I negotiated for free audiovisual aids, convention hall facilities, and a suite for my family.

Although the seminars were successful, finding a reliable and likable travel agent to help with our needs was a chore. Every year we contracted with a different agency because each turned out to be inefficient and charged too much commission. One year, as I was about to fire the owner of a local agency, I met Lazz, the lady in charge of his convention sales.

She was pleasant, efficient, and anxious to please. At the course in Hawaii, there were many compliments. The day before the course ended, I saw her at the pool and we chatted over a mai tai. I told her I was very pleased with her performance and asked her if she would be interested in working with us next year. She wanted to but warned me that she might not be with her current boss. She wanted to start her own agency. I told her that I wanted her to be our travel agent. Jokingly I said, "If you go out on your own and need any backing, let me know."

We all returned home, getting back into our normal hectic lifestyles. I had temporarily forgotten about Lazz. Two months later, she called to tell me that she was opening her own agency. "Is your offer still good?" she asked. I quickly answered that I was a man of my word and we agreed to meet for lunch and work out the details.

In a few short days, we had decided to use my money and her expertise. In a couple of years, she would be an equal partner in what we envisioned would be a very successful travel agency. In a few months it opened. Between all of our friends in the area and my yearly course, we grew to four full-time employees and a great location in El Rancho.

Medical education has been very good to me. It was very rewarding to put together a successful seminar that was financially worthwhile and medically stimulating to the participants. Well over ninety percent of our participants each year gave outstanding reviews about the course. This was the greatest compliment of all. I made a good salary from the course as the chairman and the travel agency did well. Although we worked hard for four hours a day, we had a nice vacation too. The best vacations I've ever taken have combined work with pleasure. That way I didn't get bored.

These courses have provided their share of laughs and thrills. One year I invited a dentist to give a talk on athletic injuries to teeth. Since he was a newcomer to the course, I attended his lecture to check on his performance. He did a great job and was funny, too. He emphasized that if a person got a chipped tooth in athletic competition, he should find the piece and be seen by a dentist immediately.

The next day a course faculty member was out enjoying a game of tennis with his wife. During a heated point she ran back to hit an overhead shot and chipped her husband's tooth. Having just learned about the appropriate treatment, the players got down on all fours until they located this small piece of enamel. They rushed to the nearest phone and promptly called our resident dentist, who was by the pool sunning himself. When told of this recent sports injury he replied, "Throw the chipped piece in the garbage and I'll look at the tooth tomorrow morning at breakfast."

Another year a group of faculty members decided to go fishing off the coast of Maui. When they returned several hours late to a cocktail reception, they seemed uptight. It turned out that their boat had sunk about five miles off the coast. They had been close to drowning because of high winds and waves. Had it not been for a large vessel passing by, they would have all perished. They lost their wallets, glasses, keys, and other personal belongings.

There were plenty of negatives in running the seminars too. Most years there were about twenty faculty members with whom to contend. It was a political nightmare. A neurosurgeon friend of mine and the world's nicest guy gave talks that were instructional but were less than stimulating. I asked him back each year because he knew the routine and he always got his outline in on time. But one of his partners always asked me, "Why don't you ever ask me to your course? Don't you think I can lecture?"

One of the cardiologists at Bayview Hospital wouldn't even speak to me because each year I invited his associate, the chief of cardiology, who gave very informative talks. The head of medical education at the hospital frequently ignored me because each year the hospital put on a sports medicine conference that failed miserably while our course, year after year, received a positive national response.

If someone didn't perform up to standards or their reviews were continually bad, I had an obligation to replace them. It was hard to tell a close friend that he or she needed to be replaced. One year I promised the faculty members I would send them a copy of their evaluations. That was a mistake. Two of my close friends gave the most boring talks and presented the worst slides imaginable. I purposely did not send them their evaluations, but sensing their poor performance, they asked to see them. Since then neither they nor their wives have spoken to me.

It was fun but I've had enough. I have nothing to prove anymore. I ran a successful course for seven years and have never lost a dime.

People attended my seminars from as far away as Canada, Florida, Bermuda, and Yugoslavia. I got tired of creating enemies over this course. It was very difficult to tell close friends that their outlines were incomplete, their slides were too dark, or their lectures weren't stimulating. I got sick of doctors avoiding me because my course was more successful than theirs or I hadn't asked them to lecture. I had begged long enough for faculty to get their overdue outlines to me. You have to know when to say when.

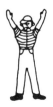

33. Fourth Down and Goal

WHAT WAS I going to do? I needed to change my practice. I needed to change my life. It was time to consider the ultimate orthopedic practice. One aspect of practice that bothered me the most was the Hopeless Health Plan. Thirty percent of my patients belonged to this miserable insurance plan. It had caused me so much grief that I asked to meet with their management.

My office manager and I met with an administrator to present proof of written authorizations for surgeries performed on patients which had not been paid. My contract guaranteed payment within forty-five days of service and several of these accounts were a year or two old. He was embarrassed and said the bills would be paid promptly. We waited two months without payment. I phoned the medical director and told him that if I didn't have a check on my desk by 5:00 p.m., I would send bills to all the patients. He said that he was sorry, but that was against the terms of my contract and I might suffer disciplinary action. I replied that it was against my contract to not be paid. Of course no check arrived and I mailed bills to all the patients.

The patients were outraged. I told them that the Hopeless Health Plan was bankrupt and it would be in their best interest to get other insurance coverage immediately, before they were left without any at all. Calls from angry patients loaded the switchboard at the health plan as patients cancelled their policies. As expected, I was terminated from the plan. I was delighted. Other doctors in town, who had been illegally dropped from the plan, followed me in filing lawsuits. I was a pied piper when it came to medical lawsuits.

Speaking of litigation, my case against Dr. Small for refusing to hire me at the university clinic finally went to trial after a wait of two years. Depositions were taken as the university tried desperately to build a defense diminishing Dr. Small's anti-Semitism. His deposition helped me considerably, as he lost his composure when asked about not wanting to hire a Jew. The defense team then persuaded the judge to agree that the trial was not about anti-Semitism, but about due process. Okay. I could live with that.

It was the defense's contention that I had been considered for the position at the university clinic but that Dr. Small's partners were better qualified. But when the defense counsel learned about Dr. Ley's inappropriate referrals in the emergency room and Dr. Baldi's failing the Boards, they decided on a different tactic. If I had been so sure that I was getting the runaround in 1984, why hadn't I filed a suit then? They claimed the statute of limitations had run out. The defense floundered again when their own prize witness, Dr. Quackmont, took the stand and admitted that as late as 1986 he had encouraged me to wait.

Dr. Stalin was then put on the stand to testify that he hadn't met me before 1984. But my attorney asked him to read a note I had written in 1983, thanking him for taking me to lunch and discussing the arthroscopy equipment at the hospital. He admitted that that lunch meeting had slipped his little mind. He said he had made phone calls to Flatville, had gotten negative reports about me, and that was the reason I didn't receive privileges at the university. But my attorney asked him why these people weren't deposed or brought to trial. He said he didn't know. Next witness.

Things were looking mighty grim for their side, so they brought up the big cheese himself, the incomparable Dr. Small. He told the jury that his selection of his own partners was a coincidence and that he had nothing against me personally. He added that he didn't recall my ever asking for privileges. He didn't even know I was interested. The jury was so disgusted that they started looking at me and rolling their eyes. I knew then that it was over.

The defense made one last effort. They flashed my yearly earnings on a huge screen in the courtroom, which showed the jury that I made four times the income of any doctor in Dr. Small's group. My attorney pointed out that this meant I was four times better than any orthopedist in their group. I noticed the jurors giggle.

And finally, victory! The jurors were out half a day and then decided. The verdict was unanimous. Dr. Small and his cohorts were guilty on twenty counts. I was awarded $200,000. I turned and smiled at Dr. Small. His wife wept as the verdict was read. On the way out of the courtroom he shouted at me, "You're an asshole." What a sore loser. As soon as their appeal is over, antitrust litigation will be filed against Dr. Small. I just hope he stays alive long enough to take another whipping.

I later interviewed the jury members. They all felt that Dr. Quackmont was lying, that Dr. Stalin was a hired gun, and that Dr. Small was the epitome of a very little man with a Napoleon complex. They agreed that I didn't even need to testify. I could have gotten the same results by just putting those doctors on the stand.

I turned my attention to revamping my practice. The less insurance we billed, the fewer write-offs we took. No more charging a patient $80 for an office visit and accepting $52 as payment in full. I knew that I would lose about thirty percent of my business with this newfound attitude, but I would replace the loss with medical-legal exams. This involves examining patients who have been in auto accidents. The whole process takes about twenty minutes and can be billed at $600 or more.

The companies pay in full and we don't send out the reports unless we receive payment. The insurance companies and attorneys have no problem with this as they know they have no case without this information. If the patient doesn't show up for the examination, we charge a no-show fee that is always paid.

The best parts of medical-legal work are depositions and testifying in court. The hourly rate for depositions is $500, and we receive $2,000 for a half day in court, paid in advance. But there's more to life than money.

Another major source of stress I wanted to avoid in perfecting my practice was operating on hospitalized patients. First, in orthopedic surgery, a lot of this work is total joint replacement in elderly people. There are many problems with these cases. The surgery is scheduled to start at 7:30 a.m. and usually gets underway about 8:30 a.m. This is due to the anesthesiologist moving along at a snail's pace.

Second, older patients have a multitude of postoperative complications, like embolisms to their lungs and brains. Yes, in surgery, sooner or later, we all have complications. But elderly people have more than usual and the doctor has very little control over this.

Third, the number of phone calls I get on inpatients is discouraging —about three to four calls a day. Most of them are from the utilization review committee, which wants to know how much longer I need to keep the patient in the hospital, because her insurance company is starting to make noise. My reply is usually, "That woman just had her hip replaced two days ago and hasn't even gotten out of bed yet." The nurses and physical therapists call often, too.

Last, I send a bill to Medicare for $3,500 for the privilege of being held up in surgery, making rounds on the patient every day for two weeks, getting numerous phone calls daily, and dodging complications, and I receive a grand total of $1,875. That's right. That's what we're willing to accept as physicians because we have no say in the rules or the figures. If you don't like it, lump it.

So what's the answer? You guessed it. Don't do any more hospital work than is absolutely necessary to maintain your privileges and do everything else on an outpatient basis. The Surgicenter is run by doctors, for doctors. The cases start on time and the turnover time between cases is about ten minutes. The hassle is virtually nonexistent. I bill $2,500 for a fifteen-minute knee case and get about eighty-five to one hundred percent of the fee. There are no patient rounds and I almost never get a phone call. The patients do well and are happy. Why ever set foot in a hospital unless you have to?

The physical therapy businesses were incredibly successful. They generated well over $2 million for me, but I noticed recently that some problems were beginning to surface. More and more legislation was being passed that would soon make it illegal for doctors to send their patients to facilities in which they had a financial interest. It was just a matter of time.

In addition, our contracting therapist was accused of "billing errors" for services he did not render. And some patients complained that one of the male therapists was not being professional during massage treatments. I brought up this concern to the therapist on three occasions and he denied it. But I knew the accusing patients. They were reliable and I was feeling very uneasy about this.

The problems were mounting. It was time to sell. The numbers looked good and our reputation was decent. Dr. Gold and I decided to test the market for selling the Bayview practice. It sold for $500,000. The El Rancho practice sold for $200,000. Two more headaches gone.

Another reason to limit your practice is the liability. Patients no longer place doctors on a pedestal and they are clearly inclined to sue. Polls have shown this. Many malpractice suits come from doing high-risk surgeries, like operating on indigent people or performing large surgeries such as back operations. Since my residency I have paid nearly $500,000 in malpractice premiums. And I'm a good doctor. I work hard to take good care of my patients. But I'm not God.

I operated on a young female who developed a postoperative arthroscopy infection. As I had been taught to do by defense attorneys, this was clearly noted in the records as a possible complication. Independent doctors reviewed the case and said the appropriate standard of care was well maintained. But my insurance attorney suggested we settle the case because the patient's offer was far less than what it would cost to defend the case in court. But wait a minute. I didn't cause the infection. I didn't spit in the wound. I should have.

Another man had a large tumor pressing on his sciatic nerve, causing his leg to go numb. I was immediately suspicious and tried to refer the case to another doctor. But the patient wanted me because I had been personally recommended. I clearly documented in the chart that he could sustain nerve damage from the surgery. But by removing this tumor, which had significant malignant potential, we could save his life. He had some slight nerve dysfunction following surgery, some of which was present before the operation. He sued me. His attorney stated that even though it was written in the chart in black and white, the patient claimed I never informed him of possible nerve damage. Who would you believe? I'm a physician. He's a used car salesman. Time will tell. Besides, when I think of all the cash I've paid in malpractice insurance over the past twelve years, I'm glad I've had a few lawsuits to get my money's worth.

As I look back over my short career in medicine, I realize that I may have caused a great deal of controversy. I got into medical school, perhaps in an unorthodox fashion, with marginal grades. I had to eat some crow starting out because I was too busy and didn't understand the politics of practice and how it can affect people who see their financial stability threatened by a newcomer in the community. It was the only time in my life I backed down, but I learned from the experience. I'm happy that I put my family and myself before my ego.

The emphasis I put on my skills is ultimately the one ace in the hole I've always had. My stint at the Free For All Clinic allowed me to perfect my arthroscopic skills, which to this day stand out among my peers.

My intense drive for honesty and integrity was challenged in Bayview. I put my trust in Dr. Quackmont, who was deceitful and wound up ashamed and poor. He couldn't make it in private practice, was fired at the All Sport Clinic, and pummeled to the bottom of the pit by accepting a position at Dr. Small's office masquerading as an orthopedic surgeon. He had to sell his home and retire to a convalescent community to die.

Perhaps my greatest source of pride, however, came from my triumph over Dr. Small. I came to Bayview and we locked horns the first day when he told me I wasn't wanted in the community. How could I come to a place with no patients and no referrals and succeed? Me against six guys? But Dr. Small was incredibly stupid and ignored my application at the university rather than face me. The scene in that courtroom told the story and this pathetic little man was sentenced to hang with his family watching. His supporting cast helped. Dr. Stalin's arrogant reputation helped me to establish my arthroscopic dominance quickly.

Thanks to Dr. Baldi, who helped question Dr. Small's judgment when he failed the Orthopedic Board Exams. But sending his girlfriend to spy on my physical therapy operation was the ultimate maneuver in paranoia.

I appreciated Dr. Ley moving aside to make room for me in Dr. Laddie's office. I'm sorry that I had to expose his extramarital fling, but this type of favoritism has no place in medicine. It's not fair to the patients coming into the emergency room, who deserve the best care available. The honor system was clearly violated here. He has since divorced two wives.

Dr. Ley was good for a laugh, too, like the time he complained to the county medical society because I operated on a patient he had seen. He said I had stolen the lady away from him. But an ethics committee simply asked the patient if I grabbed her by the arm out of his waiting room or said negative things about him to her. She told the committee she would have never let Dr. Ley touch her and that a close friend of hers, who had had surgery by me, had recommended me. The committee struggled to formulate a letter to tell the bad news to Dr. Ley nicely.

Finally, medicine is a business, and I'm afraid the days of being a doctor to help other people or because our fathers were doctors are sadly over. It's too hard to make a buck. Insurance companies are out to get us. We make too much money and the easiest place to cut expenses is the doctor's fee. Every surgery that is contemplated or any test that's desired now requires a second opinion.

It is almost impossible to get an unbiased second opinion in the same medical community. Too many doctors hate each other. There aren't enough patients to go around, and if one doctor sees a patient that a competitor wants to operate on, he almost always will say the procedure is not indicated or not necessary. Why put money in another's pocket? So the patient doesn't get better and the insurance company wastes another $100 getting a hostile opinion. A damn far cry from the Hippocratic Oath.

I am forever indebted to Dr. Quackmont and Mark Chump for forcing me to see the unbelievable earning capacity we have as physicians. Their refusal to accommodate me and my patient in 1984 has made me a young millionaire.